PCOS Recipes

An easy guide to learn about causes of PCOS, PCOS recipes and how PCOS diet can improve your health

By

Frederic O'Connor

Table of Content

Introduction

Women tell us that they excel in adopting a certain diet. For example, one might say that she lost weight and felt better with the Atkins low-carb diet, while another might say that a vegetarian high-carb diet works best for her. So who's right? Who's right?

Both of them are right. What works for a woman may not work for a woman?

Most popular diets have components that make them healthy or successful. Nonetheless, they have weaknesses or components that are not safe, even if they produce "efficiency" like weight loss.

We have reviewed all popular diets and recipes and a large number of medical studies on diets and recipes of PCOS. We distilled the healthiest elements from every diet and research item and developed a diet that we believe most women benefit from PCOS.

The Healthy PCOS Diet is intended to help you rebuild your health and keep your health vibrant for the rest of your life. Nothing is more important than your wellbeing. A healthy body helps you to live and be the woman that you want to be.

We refer to the essential food elements necessary to sustain life and good health. Please understand, good nutrition is as important as clean air and pure water. For your body, eating French fries is like smoking a cigarette or drinking water from the dioxin-contaminated well. In any case, you are destroying your body, endangering your health, and reducing your lifespan.

You will want to master the art of nutritious, healthy eating if you want to deal with your PCOS symptoms, have successful pregnancies, and enjoy a healthy and long life.

This book outlines diet and recipes that you can live comfortably throughout your life which also reduces PCOS symptoms and improves your overall health considerably.

The PCOS diet and recipes in this book recommends that you do not consume any processed, fabricated foods. You are overfed and undernourished. The PCOS recipes will correct this imbalance.

Chapter 1: PCOS & Diet

Follicles develop on the ovaries in each menstrual cycle. Eggs develop within those follicles, one of which reaches maturity earlier than the other and is released into the fallopian tubes. It's "ovulation." The remainder of the follicles disappears into the ovary.

But the ovaries are larger than normal for polycystic ovaries and a collection of undeveloped follicles, rather like a bunch of grapes, emerge in clumps. Polycystic ovaries are not necessarily disturbing and cannot even influence your fertility.

Nonetheless, a series of symptoms may occur if the cysts cause a hormonal imbalance. This disease sequence is considered a syndrome. These symptoms are the difference between PCOS and polycystic ovaries simply.

You can, therefore, have polycystic ovaries without PCOS. All PCOS females, however, will have polycystic ovaries. Polycystic Ovary Syndrome (POSS) is the name given to a metabolic condition in which a woman has polycystic ovaries and other symptoms that reflect imbalances in reproductive or other hormones.

1.1 What Is PCOS (Polycystic Ovary Syndrome)?

We refer to PCOS as a "metabolic" condition. By this, we mean that there are multiple components in the basic process of the body that is gone away. Since you have a single entire body, difficulty or deficiency in one region creates disease in other areas. PCOS is a dysfunction that is linked to your entire body, not just your ovaries.

PCOS presents a complex and baffling array of symptoms. Each woman with PCOS will have some combination of the following symptoms.

- Irregular or incomplete proportions.

- Infertility

- Infertility

- Acne

- Obesity or weight loss in capacity

- Excessive facial hair or body hair (hirsutism)

- Resistance to insulin and likely diabetes

- Scalp hair thinning

- Hyper pigmented velvety folds of the skin (acanthoses nigrans)

- High blood pressure

- Blood pressure

- Androgens (testosterone)

Multiple hormone imbalances, commonly including:

- Cortisol

- Estrogen

- FSH (Folic Hormone Stimulus).

- Insulin.

- LH (hormone Latinization).

- Progesterone.

- Prolactin

- Hormones of the thyroid.

How is PCOS common?

It is estimated that 4% to 10% of all women have PCOS. However, as many women are unfamiliar with PCOS or some aspect of it, the number actually probably exceeds 10%. PCOS is the most prevalent hormonal condition in women during the reproductive years. PCOS is a major infertility cause. Symptoms of PCOS often begin to appear soon after puberty.

PCOS is a threat

PCOS may but cannot be reduced to the long-term health consequences of cardiovascular disease

- Diabetes

- Diseases associated with pregnancy

- Cancer

- Symptoms of epilepsy

Below is a sample of what PCOS and your health have to say in the medical studies.

There is regular evidence of pancreatic fatigue in PCOS patients. The resistance to insulin usually forces the pancreas to overwork to secrete lots of insulin. This leads to cellular dysfunction, an inability to produce enough blood sugar insulin, and diabetes.

- 40% of women with PCOS have abnormal levels of blood sugar, and 10% have type 2 diabetes.

- In adolescents with PCOS, the incidence of diabetes is similar to that seen in adults.

- Women with PCOS have imbalances of blood sugar at rates that are as high as those in the world's highest-risk ethnic groups, such as Pima Indians.

- PCOS, irrespective of weight, is associated with high LDL "poor" cholesterol.

- Together, PCOS and obesity contribute to consistently elevated triglycerides that cause cardiac disease.

- In women with PCOS, high blood pressure is commonly seen.

- PCOS is related to cardiovascular disease symptoms such as increased development of blood clots, increased swelling, and thickening of blood vessel walls, elevated cholesterol, and triglycerides.

- 77% of people with abnormally rare or poor menstrual flux have PCOS proof, and 33% have elevated blood sugar levels.

- The clinical analysis of nurses found a 2.2-fold increase in the risk of type 2 diabetes progression using a 40-day or more menstrual period length as a measure. The study also showed an increase of 53 percent of cardiovascular disease events in irregular measles.

- Women with PCOS report hormonal disorders, including elevated gestational diabetes, hypertension caused by breastfeeding, and pre-eclampsia, for both obese and non-obese women. Preeclampsia may develop in late pregnancy, with a sudden rise in blood pressure, excessive weight gain, generalized swelling, urinary protein, severe headache, and visual disturbances.

- People with PCOS also have an increased risk of endometrial cancer. The risk of ovarian cancer is 2.5 percent, especially among women who have never used oral contraceptives. The risk of breast cancer with PCOS is not significantly increased.

- Women with seizure disorders are exposed to increased PCOS risk.

As you can see, you don't want to neglect PCOS. "Watchful waiting" isn't the best choice for you.

Is it possible to treat PCOS by diet?

Dietary, exercise, and lifestyle improvements are essential methods for dealing with PCOS.

Just 7% –10% weight loss in many women will lead to regular cycles of ovulation. An important part of a successful weight loss scheme is a healthy diet.

Several recent research has shown that a calorie-restricted diet helps to normalize hormones, induce ovulation, boost fertility, and minimize other PCOS problems. Whether a "best" diet for PCOS is low in fat and low in carbon is not clear; studies show that either diet can work as long as calories are small.

The issue with a calorie-restricted diet is that long-term maintenance is difficult. Another problem with the use of these restricted diets is that women with PCOS have a deteriorated satiety mechanism, according to a recent study. In other words, for PCOS women, it may be more difficult to feel that they've eaten enough. Impaired satiety makes staying in an artificially reduced-calorie diet twice difficult.

1.2 What Causes PCOS?

There is little consensus on what causes PCOS and no inference.

- Genetic predisposition is the most common reason offered for PCOS.

- Overproduction of insulin, addiction to insulin, and obesity.

- Petrochemical environmental pollution.

PCOS can also have possible additional underlying causes:

- Drug adulteration

- Autoimmune diseases.

- Chronic swelling.

- Certain medicines.

If you change your diet, some of the factors causing the PCOS may be reduced or removed. You will have will the symptoms and become much happier. Most of these suggested PCOS factors can be changed by changing health.

The majority of experts believe that polycystic ovary syndrome is, at least partly, caused by a set of genes from which you were born.

PCOS is partly a Genetic Disorder

Your inherited makeup is a little different from women without PCOS. 7 8 for example, a study recently performed on the ovarian DNA of people with or without PCOS at Nanjing Medical University. PCOS ovaries were distinct to those in normal ovaries. Some of these genes were activated when they should not have been active, some of which were inactive. Faulty genes contribute to cell instability and irregular metabolism.

Genetic Predisposition

Many women with PCOS have been told that their condition is genetically inheritable and that nothing can be done except to take birth control pills to minimize symptoms. Most people believe that genes are defined by the characteristics of your body, how you act, which conditions (or not) you get, and how long you live. It's a theory.

You are not "doomed" born to a result you have no power over. Your fate for safety is not set. Recent research has completely discredited "genetic determinism."

Genetic research has shown that your characteristics or traits are not cast into stone forever when you are conceived. Alternatively, their behavior is influenced by climate. Of examples, imagine your mother had taken DES (synthetic estrogen) while you were on her womb. The essence of the atmosphere will have a major influence. Your doctor would have given you DES to deter mistake or to have a healthy pregnancy and a healthier baby. You'd be born as a seemingly healthy baby. And, due to subtle changes in the cellular environment, you would have had a significantly higher risk of reproductive tract deformities and anomalies including a rare form of vaginal cancer, put in when the DES chemistry came through.

Speak of your genetic blueprint as "pencil written." In this case, DES was like a large eradicator that erased and replaced part of your blueprint with another blueprint. The same applies to everything else in your environment, from conception to death. You are continually under the control of your environment, inside or outside the body.

You can't change what happened to you already. If your mom takes DES, cigarettes smoked, drinks alcohol, and eats a lot of fried food while you are in her womb, you're a different person than if she didn't do that.

You have a lot of life control, and so can have a big impact on your genetic strategy.

One such control mechanism is your diet.

We speak of our height as set in stone genetically. While the standard of diet varies, entire populations change. Since World War II, the average height of Japanese adults and women has increased almost six inches. Why? Over the years, their diet has changed dramatically, leading to physical changes that were previously unchangeable by many people.

A single woman's genetic blueprint can form her with rounded hips, backrests and thighs, and delicate breasts with delicate shoulders. This basic form can be lived in at 135 or 195 pounds depending on diet choices, with important differences in its day-to-day experience and long-term health.

Also important is that you are genetically and biochemically unique to anyone else. For many women, a "one size fits all" diet won't work. So what you eat will affect you differently.

Example: Health authorities told you to reduce your salt intake if your blood pressure is high. However, studies show that only 30% to 50% of people can reduce their blood pressure by reducing their intake of salt. Salt restriction does not reduce other people's blood pressure.

Your current genetic blueprint will determine if your blood pressure is reduced by salt restrictions.

Diet and Food Adulteration

The flavor, smell, or quality of your drug is enhanced by hundreds of additives and other ingredients. While these chemical additives are licensed by the FDA, they are not safe for use.19 a family of substances known as excitotoxins is the most important example, which are chemical substances that damage nerve cells. They stimulate nerve cells to fire so quickly that they are exhausted and may die.

The nerve cells in the brain area known as hypothalamus are, unfortunately, extremely sensitive to excitotoxins. Hypothalamus is a group of specialized cells that mainly link the endocrine (glandular) with your brain's nervous systems. In the hypothalamus, nerve cells control the hypothesis by producing chemicals that either stimulate or suppress hormone secretions from the hypothesis.

Therefore, if your hypothalamus damages the nerve cells, your body will be impaired to maintain a balanced hormone.

Some excitotoxins, such as glutamate, aspartate, and cysteine, are normal. Others, like MSG, are man-made. MSG, a very popular flavoring ingredient, is a glutamate and sodium mixture. For mice, a decrease for LH (luteinizing hormone) and GH (growth hormone) was caused by high MSG doses. Low doses of MSG, on the other hand, have shown an abnormally high LH level. Elevated LH is one of PCOS women's main reproductive issues.

Administration of MSG in rats, when very young, significantly reduced ovarian and hyperphysical weights, demonstrated an absence of or affecting the cyclicity of the ovary during puberty, and had significantly higher levels of serum prolactin. Some human excitation tests also lowered the amounts of Luteinizing hormone (LH), follicle-stimulating hormone (FSH) and estrogen. It is sometimes referred to as "vegetable protein" or "plant protein" on food labels. HVP is derived from an acid and caustic soda-treated plant material. The material includes glutamate, aspartate, and cystoic acid, which are all excitotoxins.

Most products, including meats, frozen foods, cereals, fruit, sauces, soups, and dressings for salads, include HVP. HVP is present in many items. Be aware that only' vegetable protein' or' plant protein' may be labeled. "Vegetable protein," if it isn't really, may seem like something that is really healthy.

When your mother was pregnant with you, excitotoxins could have been adversely affected by your developing hypothalamus, which would lead to long-term reproductive problems when you became an adult. You can see the brain when "hard-wired" as you develop from an embryo. Your mother might have disrupted the "heat" of your brain accidentally-and indefinitely-by eating excitotoxins or being subjected to toxic chemicals and hormones.

Excitotoxins and other food additives have a significant effect on your health and your unborn children's future health. For a fact, they seem to lead to the effects of your PCOS.

Diet and autoimmune disease

Other autoimmune diseases have been reported to affect fertility. It is not yet clear whether PCOS causes these conditions. Autoimmune disease is an inflammatory condition in which your immune system mistakenly attacks your body's organs or other tissue, thinking it's' foreign' to your body.

Some of these causes tend to contribute to autoimmune diseases:

- Sex–almost 79% of US 8.5 million patients with autoimmune diseases are women.

- Estrogen, progesterone, testosterone, prolactin, growth hormone, and insulin-like growth factor-1 (IGF-1) disorders or alterations to hormones, not limited to Genetic predisposition inherited.

- Environmental considerations-food, water, air, and physical objects and microorganisms. Biological influences such as food, toxic metals, contaminants, bacteria, medicines, you call them something.

All of these factors affect the immune system. There are many autoimmune conditions, and there is no simple cause.

Link between Hashimoto's Disease and PCOS

A recent medical report has shown a link between PCOS and Hashimoto's, which is autoimmune thyroiditis.

To reproductive health and reproduction, a healthy thyroid gland is important. Inflammatory disorder, the immune system attacks and destroys the thyroid gland. Therefore, if you have Hashimoto's syndrome, you will have pregnancy complications such as infertility much more often. Sufficient thyroid hormone development is also required for proper fetal and neonatal growth and growth. The study has found that 27 percent of PCOS women have elevated thyroid antibodies to just 8.3 percent of the control group. Elevated antibodies indicate an infectious, activated immune system. PCOS patients also have higher levels of TSH than non-PCOS people, indicating that PCOS thyroid has not gained the same level of success in generating sufficient thyroid hormones.

Thyroid ultrasound showed that 42.3 percent of PCOS women have normal pictures of autoimmune thyroiditis (Hashimoto's disease), but only 6.5 percent of controls.

Link Entre Autoimmunity und PCOS

In a further recent study performed by 108 people with menstrual cycle disruptions, PCOS, endometriosis, or chronic ovulating disease, researchers found that 40 percent had immune auto-immunity antibodies compared with only 14percent for women without one of that conditions 40.

PCOS–Autoimmune Connection-C-Reactive Protein?

CRP (C-reactive protein) is an infection and inflammation signal protein in the body. Women with PCOS have considerably increased CRP concentrations in comparison to women with a normal menstrual rhythm and normal androgen levels. Low-grade inflammation seems to be a characteristic of PCOS. We could speculate that an autoimmune condition is partly responsible for the inflammation.

If an autoimmune condition does not cause CRP, it may be caused by some other chronic infection or inflammation. Or it can be because of "oxidant stress," which is a condition where antioxidant defenses are depleted and inflammation caused by free radical damage to your cells.

Role of the PCOS Diet

PCOS Diet is created to help you minimize the risk of autoimmune reactions by eliminating as many inflammatory factors as possible from your food. We are also going to prescribe foods that support the thyroid function.

1.3 The Basis of the PCOS Diet

What you eat affects what your genes do. Since your chromosomes are predisposed to PCOS, you should change your diet and change what your genes do. Modified genetic variation will enhance the effects of any PCOS that you have.

We urge you to stick to your ancestral heritage and feed as your ancestors did. Since you still have your DNA, feeding as you did makes sense.

Over the past 2, 6 million years, humans and the human genome have evolved slowly. Since the advent of agriculture about 10, years ago, our genes have changed relatively little.

From the last hundred years, the diet has undergone a complete transformation with the advent of modern methods of food processing. In comparison, our lifestyle was quickly and profoundly altered around 10, years ago. Indeed, 100 years ago, most of the food products you see on the supermarket shelf today did not exist.

The disparity between what people consume and what we eat naturally has contributed to the dramatic increase in health issues. Two-thirds of Americans are overweight or obese. Some examples:

- 90 percent of the population may suffer from high blood pressure at some point in their lives

- 40% of Americans in the middle Ages have metabolic syndrome (similar to PCOS and Syndrome X).

- Seventeen million Americans suffer from diabetes and unknown pre-diabetic, much bigger numbers.

In order to manage PCOS and many other chronic diseases, we will need to change our diet. DNA can't be traded. Therefore, our best choice is to change our diet.

What Agriculture Did to Our Ancestors

Ancient hunter-gatherers have historical and archeological evidence that is lean, fit, and mainly free of signs and symptoms of chronic disease. The health of hunters who consumed lean meat, fruit, and vegetables decreased; however, when they shifted to a grain-based diet: average adult height.

- Shorter operating life.

- Higher infant mortality.

- High incidence of osteoporosis, rickets, other deficiencies of vitamins and minerals.

Numerous studies have also shown that most of our common diseases have developed, including obesity, diabetes, and cardiovascular diseases, as more recent hunter-gatherers adopt a Western diet and lifestyle.

Return to Our Dietary Genetic Roots

Our forefathers ' genetic composition is practically identical to the genes we have today. The food our ancestors needed for optimum working is, therefore, the same food we do. Our dietary requirements are similar to theirs.

Since we know that the food that influences our genes is a part of our' environment,' it's important to check what food our forefathers ate.

Your ancestors have received their food from our natural environment. Today, the natural environment is destroyed. We will have to "jump and gather" healthy foods on our local food markets, taking care to avoid all our unhealthy foods.

Basic Elements of a Healthy PCOS Diet

Calorie count or portion control is not required. Use your common sense only. The PCOS Diet is not in the modern meaning of the term "diet." It simply eats food that is helpful for optimum gene expression and avoids unhelpful food.

There is no single-size diet that fits all. The chromosomes are different from anybody else. So a food that is helpful to another person may not help you.

Eat the highest possible quality of food. Be aware of environmental pollutants in your food, and avoid them. Use as far as possible organically produced and healthy ingredients.

- All the freshwater fish, seafood, and very lean meat you want to eat if it's as healthy and contamination-free as possible.

- All the non-starchy fruit and vegetables you want can be eaten.

- Stop both kernels.

- Avoid all vegetables.

- Remove all food dried, packaged, and distilled.

PCOS Diet Conforms to Scientific Recommendations

Higher-protein, moderate-carbohydrate alternatives to PCOS diet are consistent with the 2005 National Academy of Sciences ' Institute of Medicine's updated Dietary Reference Intakes (DRI)68 To satisfy the daily energy and nutrient needs of an adult the DRI study advises 45-65% calories from starch, 10% from daily consumption, these ranges give the flexibility to plan a healthy diet.

While we disagree with certain aspects of the Government's dietary directives, we agree with the caloric distribution recommended for carbohydrates, protein, and fat.

1.4 Healthy PCOS Diet vs. Low-Carb Diet

The diets of Atkins and South Beach are one of the most common. Both are considered "low carb" diets, which means you highly recommend reducing carbon calories to lose weight.

The PCOS diet, on the other hand, is not designed specifically for weight loss, although weight loss is one of its primary benefits. It is designed to improve your health and reduce PCOS symptoms.

Food	PCOS Diet	Low-carb Diet
Protein	Moderately	
High	Moderate	
Carbohydrate	Moderate	Low
Total fat	Moderate	High
Saturated fat	Moderate	High
Monounsaturated fat	High	Moderate
Polyunsaturated fat	Moderate	Moderate
Omega-3 fats	High	Low
Fiber	High	Low
Vegetables & fruits	High	Low
Nuts & seeds	Moderate	Low
Dairy foods	None	High
Gluten grains	None	Low
Salt	Low	High
Refined sugars	None	Low
Glycemic load	Low	Low
Acid-Alkaline balance	Balanced	Acid
Strict portion controls	None	Yes
Processed foods	No	Yes
Artificial food additives	No	Yes

| Artificial sweeteners | No | Yes |

Similarities and variations are found here when compared the PCOS diet to a low carbon diet:

Type of carbon vs. Carb Restriction

One distinctive feature in the type of carbohydrates is permitted between the PCOS diet and several low-carb diets.

We believe it is time to go beyond simply reducing carbohydrates to lose weight. Research has increasingly shown that the carbohydrate type is as important as controlling the total intake of carbohydrates.

Johns Hopkins University conducted a 2005 study that examined the dietary intake of 572 people a full year.[69] Bodyweight was found to equate with the glycemic index of the ingested carbohydrates. The glycemic index is a glycemic response measure of the ingestion of various types of carbohydrates. The higher glycemic index is tended to be refined or processed carbohydrates, whereas the whole carbohydrate has a lower glycemic index. The higher the glycemic index of consumed carbohydrates, the higher the tendency to add weight.

The study also found that there is no connection between weight and total daily consumption of carbohydrates or the percentage of total carbon calories. In other words, whether people were on a low-carb or high-carb diet was irrelevant.

This study shows that carbohydrate type is extremely important for the control of weight. Clearly, the sort of carbohydrate you use is critical to your overall health, not just your weight.

Chapter 2: PCOS Diet Levels

2.1 The PCOS Diet:

- Recommended level

- Maintenance level.

You can choose the degree that suits you best.

Recommended level

The recommended level of the diet is designed to assist you:

- Reduce PCOS symptoms such as resistance to insulin

- Lose weight of fat

- Enhance your fertility

- Boost your basic health and vitality

- Boost your lifespan

The recommended food levels are much more restricted than food products at the maintenance level.

Healthy diet for PCOS and remain at that level for at least one month. You can stay for no maximum time at the recommended level – you can remain there for several years, several months, or the rest of your life.

You just eat foods on the "healthy ingredients" list at the recommended level. But if you don't want to or cannot restrict yourself to "Great Foods," sometimes foods on the "Better Foods" lists may be used.

Maintenance Level

The replacement is a more flexible diet, allowing you to choose a larger range of foods that maintains a healthy diet for most people. At the maintenance level, you eat mostly from the list of best foods, but sometimes you add food from the list of good foods.

You will decide whether you are going to continue at the recommended level or to switch to the maintenance level after at least one month at the recommended level. Each woman is unique in biochemistry and genetics. You may need to remain at the minimum level for the rest of your life, or in one month or two; you may switch to the maintenance level.

When you go to a Maintenance level, and your symptoms or weight tend to increase, go down to the recommended level and stay there until you get the health outcomes you're looking for before you try to switch to Maintenance again.

Food Lists

The balanced PCOS diet classifies food in each major food group as great, decent, and not good.

Lists with the best foods. Food on these lists will give you the best health outcomes possible. You will only eat food on this list as long as you are at the prescribed diet level.

Good food charts. Good food list. You can eat foods occasionally on the Good Food Lists if your diet is maintained. For the average person, these foods are relatively healthy. However, some of them can lead you back. We cannot predict whether certain foods on the good list will benefit you, have no effect, or cause problems for all women. Each of the women is unique.

Try not to substitute food from the best lists for foods from the good lists. A good list of foods can be consumed on special occasions or from time to time. They are not the core of your diet every day.

Lists include nutritious or perhaps unhealthy foods. Many foods on these lists may not be appropriate for some women, but those lists should not be eaten for some other foods. When you are dealing with PCOS, obesity, weight, and general health, keep these things in mind.

Each woman is unique

There is significant genetic variation among women with PCOS. To achieve results, some will have to be permanently at the recommended level. Others can move relatively quickly to the maintenance level. Others are going to be somewhere between.

You will have to experiment in some way to determine what diet or diet mix is best for you.

Some women are slim. Some women. Some of them are obese. Some are in the center. Slim people can benefit from the recommended dietary level. Another slim woman at the recommended level may not have to be at all.

The biggest challenge can be overweight women. Some are' closed' for insulin resistance in fat-building mode. Other overweight people have severe hormonal disorders causing a loss of appetite and binge consumption. Overweight women should probably be at the recommended level for a longer time. If they go to maintenance level or enjoy "bad" food, they can get into metabolic trouble.

Recommended level distractions are OK, but "the miles can differ." Some will have minor negative consequences for a diversion. For others, they look like they've got a pound if they have some bacon.

The "Recommended level" is just that not obligatory. If you want to reach a lower safety result, you can include foods at a maintenance level and, even rarely, appreciate the disallowed foods.

Exercise Is Essential – Diet Alone Is Not Enough

Keep in mind that dieting alone may not be adequate to cope with the PCOS symptoms adequately. You will also have to practice regularly. Training is an important part of your plan to normalize your hormones and rid yourself of excess weight. View the diet as your right leg and your left leg as your workout. When you try to walk on only one knee, you can't go very far or fast.

But you can go much further and faster if you use both legs. For further information on exercise.

The choice is yours

The PCOS diet is going to ask you a lot. You will be asked to revamp your diet and eating habits completely.

The result of your illness depends to a large degree on what you do–or do not. That's what you eat.

It's your medicine to eat. What "medicine" would you like to take? Who is good for you, or who is not good for you?

There is no completely simple, completely easy diet for wellbeing. You cannot go to your local supermarket, bar, or have a healthy meal that you can get into the microwave or cook in your car.

A healthy diet requires commitment, persistence, and determination. The least resistant is to eat packaged and prepared tasty foods or to follow a simple "fad" diet without any problem.

That path will inevitably lead you to cardiovascular diseases, diabetes, and many chronic conditions, which can result in early death.

The less resistant path is not the path we recommend. They propose a more challenging course to build your own food and diet plan–discarding and replacing unhealthy foods with healthy ones.

The diet we prescribe is not easy or difficult. Focus and persistence are all necessary.

Make steady progress towards a healthy diet on a daily basis.

Is it a "detrimental diet?" It could be depending on how you perceive life. As an example, would you feel "deprived" if you stopped smoking?

You may until you're not worried about it anymore and don't notice it at all. Eventually, you are delighted to quit smoking–saving money, smelling home and clothes easier, eating better, getting more strength, and reduced the risk of lung cancer considerably.

We invite you to eat the same thing.

You are accustomed to eating unhealthy foods if you are like most Americans. You're going to stop eating them on this diet. You may first feel deprived because the new foods will not provide you with a flavor or immediate boost to which you are accustomed. But you will slowly become familiar with new flavors and textures. More notably, you should start feeling better, so you're on the right track with a lot of positive improvements.

Finally, you have a serious disorder, which is difficult to treat and heal. We suggest that you use a healthier diet to control your PCOS symptoms and reduce the risk of heart disease and diabetic problems. Your lifespan is also going to be extended. Nothing to tell about being pregnant and having a child! So you've got a lot to do!

Our Pledge to You

What does success or failure mean? The diet plans basically a "good thing" way of eating. Our diet plan reflects how we were designed to eat genetically based on hundreds of thousands of years of human history.

This is not a meal, as in the diet for weight loss. It's a way of life the way we have all lived until very recently. It is normal. Normal. It is what our bodies prosper and seek. We have lived since the dawn of human history in a healthy diet and lots of physical activity.

It is a diet that is in harmony with our being. Our promise is that if you follow the guidelines outlined in this book, you will make "good things possible."

2.2 What to Eat

This book is not a diet book for weight-loss but specifies that we eat "x" g of protein, "y" g of sugars, and "z" g of fat. We're not asking you to limit yourself every day to "x" calories. Most popular diet books are approached "one size fits all." This strategy is not successful for PCOS.

People who have PCOS do not have a single problem in a homogenous population. Some of them are extremely obese, some of them very slim and somewhere between them. Some are resistant to insulin, while others are not. Many suffer from severe chronic hormonal disorders; others have a less disordered profile.

Some may eat a lot of food and not gain weight, while others even look for food laterally. Many people eat binge food, while others don't consume enough.

Many benefit from a high protein diet, while others get no results. Some do not have milk sugar metabolism enzymes; others do. Some are drugs that alter dietary needs, but not all of them. There are different types of metabolic problems in PCOS members.

In addition, your genetic pattern is unique to you. Many PCOS women are going to be somewhat different. From the evolutionary point of view, an ideal diet for your next woman is not perfect.

In every country in the world, PCOS people are found. The food types available vary widely from country to country.

And some people are persuaded that they have PCOS, but they don't. For example, some people may have insulin resistance, which creates some PCOS-like symptoms but does not meet all polycystic Ovary syndrome diagnostic criteria. These individuals may have genetic, "X syndrome," or diabetic syndrome. (They can still enjoy the healthy PCOS diet, however).

PCOS is an extremely complex set of signs and conditions, as you can understand. It is misleading to suggest that a common diet is the "right one" for you all.

Guidelines-What to Eat

The diet described in this book is a set of guidelines for food selection based on human history, medical research volumes, and many years of clinical experience.

It is up to you, in our instructions, to choose the specific foods to consume and the correct quantities to eat.

Main Dietary Components, provides you with extensive food lists. The preferable foods in each major food group will be found at the "recommended diet stage." Foods found at the "Maintenance diet level" may also be suitable if you do not experience serious PCOS symptoms.

We want you, above all, to eat the healthiest food possible. By being clean, we say as much as possible unprocessed and untouched through human hands. We can't stress this enough. It is clear that a diet high in refined foods is bad for your health, suggesting it is especially unacceptable for severe conditions such as PCOS.

There are some very severe restrictions on our instructions. For instance, at the level of the Recommend Diet, we ask you not to eat grains, beans, or milk. When you cut fruit, beans, and milk, most refined foods vanish from your diet immediately.

The missing processed foods will be replaced by vegetables, fish, poultry, meat, fruit, nuts, and seeds. Such foods provide all the calories you need. Just have a variety of such foods. If you are particularly hungry for a certain meal, have extra vegetables.

Guidelines-How much Eat

Some women need more than others to limit caloric intake. Eat meals of modest size. The food in our diet is high in fiber, so you can eat a relatively large quantity of food containing fewer calories than equal quantities of processed food.

You are using common sense. Common sense. Do not eat a large handful of nuts merely because they are on your menu if you need to lose weight. If you want your calories to be restricted, but you are very appetite, you may consume additional amounts of different vegetables from our recommended vegetable list.

2.3 What Not to Eat

Most of the food you find in a local supermarket or grocery shop. In reality, most of them will affect your health. They shouldn't be caught.

"Convenience" Foods

A food for convenience is created when an entire food is finished, heated, extracted, extracted, or otherwise processed and then combined with an unknown number and amount of chemical substances to alter its appearance, texture, shelf life, color, and general appearance.

Refined, processed food intake is obviously harmful to your health. These are also referred to as "cool" or "junk" products.

Food appeal. Most nutritional components of the food are destroyed during processing. Convenience foods are easily identified. We will almost always be found in stylish packaging like carton bags, plastic containers, or plastic wrap. Attractive shape, color, and texture are provided for the food itself.

Commodity foods can be found almost everywhere, in every market and in all fast-food outlets.

Generally, these foods have little or no nutrient value; only "empty" calories are provided. Your body should use energy and stored nutrients to digest or remove these foods and thus lose body reserves.

Foods of convenience pose more problems as they are likely to contain:

- Toxic metals, pesticides, fungicides, petrochemicals, antibiotics, hormones. Partially hydrogenated (altered) oils which disrupt cell membrane function

- Oxidized oils that cause free radical damage to cells a number of unhealthy food additives that lead to disease. Oxidized (rancid) oils that cause free radical damage to cells.

- Pathogenic microorganisms (bacteria, viruses, parasites)

- Excessive amounts of salt or sweeteners

- Genetically modified foods. Refined carbohydrates trigger spikes in blood sugar and hormone imbalances

The presence of these products creates tasty foods that you do not want to put in your mouth.

The typical US absorbs nearly 9 lbs. Every year, food chemicals and additives. It places an enormous burden on your detox. When these chemicals are not detoxified, they are stored indefinitely in your body and contributing to degenerative disease.

Regular consumption of unhealthy foods can lead to asthma, skin conditions, and headaches of migraine, gastrointestinal disorders, fatigue, nausea, insomnia, hyperactivity, and many other symptoms.

Keep completely away from highly-processed foods to better control PCOS and restore your wellbeing.

Oily, Fatty Foods

Most foods we consume contain oils and fats which are highly processed, heated, oxidized or chemically altered and which seriously impede the function of cells, contain unknown processing by-products, and are of direct damage to cells, including their DNA. The toxic oils and fats are sold "as is" or hidden in a wide range of foodstuffs.

Otherwise, sticky or fatty foods impair the metabolism in addition to their toxic effects. Recent scientific research has shown that the heart needs to work after a high-fat meal nearly twice as hard as after a high starch meal. Obesity not only interferes with the use of oxygen but also demands twice as much oxygen as protein or starch for energy breakdown. Reducing dietary fat helps increase our blood's ability to transport oxygen to all our tissues.

Sugary Foods

Apart from fats and oils, sweeteners like sugar or corn syrup are laden to most foods we eat commonly. Unbelievably, the average US consumes approximately 150-170 lbs. nearly 1/2 lb. of sweeteners per year. Per day! Per day! This may be five times the number of sweeteners a century ago.

The blood sugar fluctuations of refined carbohydrates such as white bread and breakfast cereals are responsible for their chronic hormone imbalances.

Foods to avoid lists

In the following chapters, in each of the main food categories, there are lists of specific "unhealthy" foods. These foods should be avoided.

Unhealthy foods certainly contain several foods you eat. The unhealthy foods on our lists may potentially be the center of your diet. We change your dietary habits by asking you to stop eating these foods. Please note that these foods are an important cause of your current health issues. In order to improve your health, you must first improve your diet.

For example, wheat products like bread, bagels, crackers, and cookies are on our "not eat" list. Some of these products are likely to be eaten on a daily basis.

- Can increase blood sugar higher than acceptable levels and cause an inflammatory hormonal response, as they are sugar and refined flour

- Contain oils which are oxygen-subjected and at high temperature, converting them into reactive free radicals that destroy the cells

- It contains gluten (gliadin) proteins to which you are infected.

You may be temporarily deprived, as refined grains are taken away as a staple of your diet. But we have plenty of alternatives for you. You're gradually getting used to new foods and don't care about how much a piece of bread or fresh pastry is lacking.

We understand that you are going from the known to the unknown. We ask you to change your way of life. This can be complicated. But it would not be too long before new, healthier dietary habits are established. Be patient. Be patient. Be constant. Be constant. You're going to be successful!

Chapter 3: PCOS Recipes

3.1 Basic Meals

The basic food section contains a few very versatile "basic" recipes. You will make meals for you and your family with many variations of animal protein and vegetables. We don't often have time to cook a gourmet meal. Sometimes in 15 minutes, we have to be able to fix a good meal.

Stir-Fry.

The stir-fry is one of our favorites. This is a recent example of what we have achieved with a stir-fry. It was 5:45 a day. If A family member had to leave at 7 p.m. so that dinner was provided at 6 p.m., so dinner wouldn't be too rushed for eating. But we were extremely busy and hadn't been to the food store for a couple of days. In the house, there wasn't much food. In 15 minutes, what could be created?

This is what we did. Here is what we did. On the stove, place a large non-stick pot, medium-low heat, and add three tablespoons of water and 2 or 3 olive oil tablespoons. Remove a few onions and a few garlic cloves from the pantry. Slice quickly and put in a covered skillet to medium heat.

There was a need for an animal protein. It looked in the fridge nothing was there. I looked at the fridge. Aha! Aha! Aha! A bag of frozen shrimp existed. Take four big handfuls of shrimp and drain them. Skillet covered. Our next thought was about vegetables. Looked back in the fridge the broccoli's head, 1-1/2 turkey, and half a Chinese chop.

We usually have plenty of veggies on hand, but that's all we had today. Sliced everything and put it in a sealed bowl. When we let it cook for one or two minutes, we decided to add some tamari (a sauce without wheat), leaving the skillet uncovered. Some discrepancies were over, but we finally added 1-2 teaspoons of turmeric for added flavor and color.

We applied a splash of more water as it appeared a little cold. We cooked the stir-fry until most of the ingredients were tender. Around 6:00 pm, we began dinner right on time.

Soups and Stews.

Tasty homemade stews and soups are quite versatile. Heartful homemade soups or products. It is a giant soup bowl or stew.

One source is chicken soup. First, we should boil a whole chicken, cut all cooked meat, and place it in a large pot of water/chicken broth. Then we cut a lot of vegetables. We normally use any veggies on hand. We don't bother to follow a recipe we're just making it as we go.

We can add 3-6 different vegetables to the soup in different amounts, depending on the type and what we had in our pockets. We cut it up and put it in the pot and let it all steam. Of course, depending on our mood, we add a considerable amount of herbs and spices.

When cooked, we can run approximately 1/3 of the soup through a mixer and put it into the pot. It makes a creamier soup. We now have a warm, protein-free soup loaded with vegetables that are both chunky and creamy in texture.

Or, we can just throw 2 or 3 fillets of chopped fish (or chunks of leftover cooked turkey) or a cheap cut of beef in the place of boiling a chicken. Our soups are not always creamed.

All we end up with is a pretty big soup bowl. It could last us one pot for a week, depending on how often we have it.

Our soups aren't watery and thin. These are rich and tragic because they have a large proportion of animal protein and vegetables. One pot is overflowing this soup. We look over-full with two plates. A high-protein soup may be a full meal, or a smaller portion may be eaten as part of a meal.

In the next few days, we ice anything we won't use. We place it in individual plastic containers in meal size and freeze it. We now have a super-fast meal to enjoy at any moment.

After we have finished eating some unfrozen soup or broth, we take 1-2 cups out of the condom and place them in the refrigerator so that they get thawed out slowly and are available at all times for "instant" dinner. We get a cup from the refrigerator anytime we feel tired or rushed, place it on a ceramic bowl, and microwave it. We've got a meal in 5 minutes now.

Salads

Salads are flexible and simple, too. In the refrigerator, we normally have some leftover beef, poultry, or fish. We simply take some lettuce, spinach, or other greens out of the fridge, wash them (if not washed yet), cut them or tear them, and put them in a bowl of salad. For that, we can add any crunchy stuff like celery or sliced calcareous. We also add any accent vegetables, such as green onions or parsley, to our hands.

Then we add our animal protein, cut or sliced. If we have no seafood, poultry, or red meat on hand, we can cook a few eggs easily and make an egg salad.

Finally, we should drizzle a dressing of salad over the plate, then blend or gently swirl the salad. We use one of the sauces and dressings in the recipes section.

We also add raw salad cashews, walnuts, or some other nut or seed in order to finish it. In about 10 minutes we can normally make a nice salad.

Sandwiches and Roll-ups

From now on, you may have found that no bread is permitted on a healthy PCOS diet. This does not mean sandwiches, toast, and jam. These are modern foods that may not be well matched to your genetic make-up. You could imagine that since the dawn of history, the sandwich has been around. This is not the case, though.

By contrary to what you might have read, by 1765, the Earl of Sandwich did not invent the sandwich. The first sandwich was recorded by the renowned rabbi, Hillel the Elder, who lived in the 1st century B.C. He started the practice of Passover sandwiching with bitter herbs, a combination of chopped nuts, apples, spices, and wine between two matzohs.

Thick blocks of coarse stalked bread, known as trenchers, were used for plates in the middle Ages. Meat and other foods have been stacked on top of the bread to be consumed with fingers and sometimes with knives. The thick and dense trenchers consumed the water, fat, and sauces. At the finish, one ate the trencher or, if starvation had been satisfied, threw his dogs into the gravely-soaked bread or gave it to a less fortunate person.

English woman Elizabeth Leslie brought the sandwich to America in 1840. She had a recipe for ham sandwiches in her cookbook, Directions for Cookery, which she suggested as a main dish. We have since adopted the sandwich as the staple of our diet. So for fewer than two decades, the sandwich has been with us. Even today, most people in the world don't usually eat sandwiches.

But since there is no sandwich bread in the healthy PCOS diet, what can you use instead? We recommend that you make "roll-ups" with wraps.

Wraps consist of any food permitted in which other foods can be wrapped. Examples of the possible wrap are:

- Salad leaves

- Leaves of chops (lightly steamed)

- Leaves of collar (lightly damped)

- Steamed slices of eggplants.

- Pickled leaves of the vine.

- Small omelets. Thin omelets.

- Sheets of Nori seaweed.

- Slices of meat.

- Leathers of vegetables.

There are several types of wrapping methods:

- Enchilada type-flats lie wrapper, spread with 2-3 filling teaspoons, fold wrapper over filling, and roll up tightly.

- Burrito style–smooth, spread filling wrapper, fold 1/4-1/3 of the path inwards, fold over filling wrapper, fold into a compact package.

- Tostada style-plate-free wrapper spread with vegetables, sprouts, meats, topping.

So you can have something similar to a sandwich. You need something other than toast.

Serving Sizes Please note that in the following recipes, the number of servings varies from one receipt to the next. We can't know how many people your family has, so please change recipes to the number of people you feed and the number of residues that you want to make.

Therefore, the size of the serving, which works well for you, can be too much or too little for another woman. Defining the proportion of meal servings is up to you. The serving sizes are only specific recommendations in each recipe.

Although some PCOS women are overweight and resistant to insulin, others are lean and insulin-resistant. We can't tell you the exact portion sizes you should eat all are unique. In fact, though, most people eat more than they need.

If you are on a Weight Control plan and have a limited number of calories you can use, you can use a vast number of online calorie counters to calculate the calorie content of any meal in this text.

Basic Meals Recipes

Basic Garden Salad

- 1/2 cup broccoli, small spears
- 1/2 cup bean sprouts
- One stalk celery, chopped
- One carrot, diced, shredded or thinly sliced
- 1-2 green onions, cut into 1" pieces
- 1/4 cup pine nuts
- 1/2 cup watercress, broken into 1" pieces
- 1/2 cup jicama, sliced
- 1/3 cup radish, thinly sliced

Note: You may select any other vegetables from the recommended list or delete them.

Basic Soup

- 1 cup string beans, chopped into 1" pieces
- 1/2 cup fresh parsley
- Two zucchinis, chopped
- Two cloves garlic
- One medium onion
- One tablespoon extra-virgin olive oil
- 2 quarts' low-salt chicken broth
- Two chicken breasts, bone, and skin removed
- Two carrots

- six tomatoes (24 ounces canned tomatoes if fresh not available) and 1/2 tablespoon turmeric Pinch of pepper (optional)

In a soup pot, add in a little olive oil, garlic, and onion. Add water and bring to a boil. Stir in chicken. Simmer in for 30 minutes. Cut, cool, and dice the chicken. Season with vegetables and spices. Simmer 15-20 more minutes. When chicken is cooked, return the chicken to the pot and serve.

Variation: Replace the chicken with a de-boned turkey breast, or 16–24 oz. Of whatever meat or fish. Add or replace any other Recommended List vegetables, if you wish.

Basic Stew

- 3/4 cup carrots, sliced

- 4 stalks celery, sliced

- 1-pound stew meat, cut into 1-inch cubes

- One teaspoon salt

- Five cloves garlic crushed one bay leaf

- One tablespoon dried thyme leaves

- 1/2 teaspoon ground pepper

- 3/4 cup chopped onion

- 32 ounces' beef or chicken stock 1/2 cup chopped parsley

- One medium-large tomato

- 1/4 cauliflower or cabbage

- Two tablespoons extra virgin olive oil

- 1 pound mushrooms (any type), sliced 3 cups pure water

Season with salt and pepper to taste. Heat up to medium-heavy kettle or crockpot, then add two tablespoons of water and two tablespoons of oil to the pan. Steam the beef until it has browned, about 8 minutes. Add all other ingredients except parsley. Simmer for several hours, and serve with chopped parsley sprinkle.

Notes: From our recommended lists you can substitute other meats, poultry or vegetables.

Basic Stir Fry

- 1/3 cup pine nuts

- 4 cloves garlic, chunks

- Two tablespoons tamari

- 1/3 Chinese cabbage, sliced

- 1 cup water or stock 1/2-pound bean sprouts

- 1/4 cup olive oil

- Four carrots, chopped

- 2 cups tender snow pea pods

- 1-2 small Japanese eggplant or 1/4 regular eggplant, cubed one medium size bok choy, sliced crosswise

- 2 pounds' lean meat or chicken, cubed or sliced

- Two medium onions, sliced

Three tablespoons of water in a large frying pan or wok, then put the olive oil and heat. Brown meat and cut it from saucepan. Add garlic and onion. Fry until soft.

Increase heat to relatively high. Add carrots and cabbage. Sauté off for about 5 minutes. Add eggplant, pea pods, and then bok choyDrop-in for a few minutes. Remove vegetable or water stock. Add meat to saucepan. Stir and ride. Simmer on for 10 minutes. If the liquid evaporates, add additional water or stock.

Add tamari and bean sprouts. Stir and simmer 30 seconds. Garnish with pine nuts and serve

Variations: You may be using beef, pork, turkey, or fish instead of chicken. Just a meat mix, if you have them on hand, is Fine. When you are using leftover meat already cooked, don't brown it just add it three minutes before cooking is over.

The densest vegetables are often used first, then the leafy ones. If you're not fond of any of the above vegetables, seek out other types.

3.2 Meat & Seafood

Asian Flank Steak

- 1 Pound flank steak two tablespoons tamari

- One tablespoon root ginger, peeled and hacked

- 1/4 cup teaspoon olive oil

- Two clove garlic, crushed

A large heavy-duty zip-top plastic bag, combine tamari, ginger, oil, and garlic. Add bag and steak. Marinate 8 hours in the refrigerator, occasionally rotating the container. Remove bag steak. Marinade reserve for basting.

Prepare the bbq or barbecue. Place the steak on the spray-coated grill rack or broiler pan and cook on each side for 8 minutes, or to the desired degree. As you cook it, you can add reserved marinade to poultry. Cut the steak diagonally around the grain, into thin slices.

Baked Buffalo Stew

- 1 pound of stewed stew

- 1 pound of stewed beef

- One colossal carrot, split in full bunks

- One small onion, cut in large pieces
- Six bunches, cut into quarters
- Three cloves of garlic, sliced
- Three sets of celery, diced
- One green pepper, chopped
- Three cloves of garlic
- fresh ground black pepper, 1/4 teaspoon
- 1/4 teaspoon salt (optional)
- One teaspoon salt-free all-purpose seasoning*
- 1/2 cup of bovine
- One teaspoon fresh horseradish(optional)

Square meat cubes in a large casserole dish. Add carrot, ointment, sprout in Brussels, garlic, celery, green pepper, tomatoes, savory, and stock. Cover tightly and bake at 275 ° F in a large oven. Five hours. Before serving, sprinkle with grated horseradish.

Beef and Pepper Fajitas

- 1-pound beef steak with one tablespoon extra-virgin oil
- One medium olive oil, slice
- 1 cup green bell pepper, sliced
- 1 cup of bell pepper purple, slice
- 1 cup of red bell pepper, stripe
- 1 cup of red bell pepper, stripes
- Two medium tocchini, cut into diagonal slices
- Two sticks celery, sliced diagonally

- Two teaspoons chili POW Add olive oil, sauté onions, peppers, courgettes, and celery until the onions are translucent.

Heat a large skillet over medium-high heat. Add olive oil and sauté onions, peppers, zucchini, celery, and seasonings until onions are translucent. Remove from pan and hold.

Remove the slices of beef and sauté until they are white. Put vegetables back into the saucepan and sauté until all is dry. Serve with your choice of Latin salsa* or salsa.

Beef, mushroom and Spinach Eggs

- 1/4 pound extra slender soil beef
- 1/2tab of cooked olive oil, 1/2 cup of chopped garlic
- 1/2 cup of chopped champignon
- 1/2 cup of fresh spinach, chopped
- One hard-boiled egg.
- Tamari to taste

Gray, medium heat ground beef, and garlic in olive oil. Add sliced mushrooms, basil, spinach, and tamari when the meat is nearly finished. Cook over low heat until wilted and tender to the spinach. Place a sliced hardboiled egg on the plate and top with it.

Beef or Buffalo Chili

- One extra virgin tablespoon
- 1/2 cup of olive oil, chopped
- 1/2 cups of celery, chopped
- 1 cup of green pepper, chopped 2-3 cloves of garlic, chopped
- 2 pounds of ground or extra maiden powder
- One teaspoon of chill powder

- 2-1/2 teaspoons of ground cumin

- Two teaspoons of dried thyme

- 1/2 teaspoon of Morton Salt Substitute or 1/2 teaspoon of regular salt. (Use approximately 16 ounces of canned tomatoes if fresh tomatoes are not available).

- Twelve ounces Chili Salsa Tomato* Wide-sprinkled heat oil.

Clean the carrots, celery, green pepper, and garlic until tender and bright (about 4 minutes). Attach the buffalo, chili powder, cumin, and thyme, then cook for 5 minutes.

In a pot, add salt, tomatoes, and Chili Tomato. Cover and cook for at least an hour at small.

Notes: You should put this dish in a crockpot. After the vegetables have been baked, add the remaining crockpot ingredients and cook for several hours.

Beef or Wild Sirloin with Mushrooms

- 1-1/2 pounds' free-range beef (or wild game) sirloins or tenderloins, visible fat removed and cut into 2x1x1 inch strips

- 1/2 cup scallions, thinly sliced

- Two tablespoons tamari

- Five tablespoons extra virgin olive oil

- Two tablespoons freshly squeezed lemon juice

- Black pepper to taste (optional)

- Two cloves garlic, minced

- Crumbled whole dried thyme leaves 1/2 teaspoon

- regular salt to taste or Morton Salt Substitute

- 1 pound Portobello mushrooms

- 1 cup rich beef stock

Remove and save mushroom stems for further use. Slice the caps nearly 1/2-inch-thick medium heat skillet up to dry. Remove two tablespoons of water and the other two tablespoons of olive oil.

Add the champagne and blend well. Sprinkle salt and pepper. Sprinkle. Cook, stirring regularly, about 5 minutes until the mushrooms are tender. Extract from the bowl the mushrooms and any liquid and set aside.

Separate bits of meat so that they don't boil when cooking Black on all sides for about 2 minutes, uncommon to medium-rare.

Place the pot over medium heat, then add about half of the meat to any marinade. Clean the water, and keep it dry. Continue with the leftover beef.

Pour out any leftover fat, leaving some browned pieces of meat. Stir well, scrape the bottom of the pot with a wooden spoon and brown it until the fluid becomes slightly thick. Reduce to medium-low heat.

Attach the beef stock to the saucepan and heat it Remove the champagne and cook while stirring for a few seconds, remove the meat and quickly cook, and repeat until the chicken is fully cooked. Serve straight away. Serve straight away.

Note: In this recipe, you can use elk, deer, antelope, or caribou beef.

Beef Sukiyaki

- 2-3 cloves garlic, minced

- 1/2 cup tamari

- Free-range chicken stock or 1-3/4 cups beef or

- Two tablespoons rice wine vinegar

- Two tablespoons beef or free-range chicken stock
- 1/2 pounds' organic or free-range flank steak
- One tablespoon olive oil
- 2 cups celery, cut in diagonal strips
- 2 cups cabbage, shredded
- 2 cups onions, sliced into thin crescents
- Swiss chard or Chinese cabbage,4 cups bok choy
- 2-5 green onions, cut diagonally
- 2 cups mushrooms, sliced
- 2-3 cups of fresh bean sprouts

Mix the garlic, tamari, vinegar and two tablespoons of stock in a sealed pan to create the marinade. Using a sharp knife, cut steak around the grain into thin slices (this is better if steak is partially frozen). Add mixture to marinade, thoroughly paint, and marinate for many hours.

Cut the vegetables and save until ready to cook. Drain the meat marinade, add the remaining 1-3/4 cup stock, and set aside for marinade. Heat wok or heavy pot, add oil. When dry, mix in meat and sauté for approximately 2 minutes until the meat starts to lose its pink color. Remove pan meat. Attach celery and onions to the saucepan, and cook for 2 minutes. Add 1/4 of the marinade, then chopping the chocolate and bok choy orchard. Brush until veggies start wilting. Put another 1/4 cup marinade in and cover with steam for 2 minutes.

Reduce heat and add wine, olive onions, and slices of beef. Disable to blend. Pour the marinade over it and put on a plate of sprouts of fresh seed.

Buffalo Burgers

- 1/2-pound ground buffalo meat

- 1/2 tablespoon horseradish
- 1/2 teaspoon Spike vegetable seasoning
- Black pepper to taste

Bring all the ingredients together and turn them into patties. Broil, barbecue, or steam-fry until finished (about 3-4 minutes per hand, or brown all over). Don't overcook them.

If needed, top with a mix of guacamole and salsa.

Creole Rabbit

- 3 pounds' rabbit meat, cleaned and cut into pieces
- One teaspoon Morton Salt Substitute or 1/4 teaspoon regular salt
- 1/4 teaspoon black pepper
- 1/4 teaspoon cayenne pepper
- 1/4 cup onion, chopped
- Three cloves fresh garlic, minced
- Two tablespoons white vinegar
- One tablespoon extra-virgin olive oil
- 1 cup sliced mushrooms
- One tablespoon fresh parsley, minced
- Two tablespoons green bell pepper, minced
- Two tablespoons green onions chopped fine
- 1/3 cup dry white wine

Wash and dry bits of rabbit, then put them in a tub. Combine salt, black pepper, cayenne pepper, onion, vinegar, garlic, and butter. Cover the bowl and marinate in the refrigerator overnight.

To oiled baking dish, switch the rabbit and marinade. Bake in 450 degrees F, preheated. Oven 1 hour. Combine remaining ingredients and pour in the rabbit over them. Bake longer than 30 to 45 minutes, until the rabbit is fork-tender.

Curried Beef Strips

- Two tablespoons extra virgin olive oil
- 4 ounces of lean beef, 1 1/4 inch strips cut
- One apple, rude
- One onion, rude
- One red pepper and rustic chopping
- 1/2 cloves of garlic, thin
- One tablespoon of curry Tamari powder for taste
- 1/2 cup water Heat pane with care. ·1/2 cup of hot water
- 1/2 cup of the pan.

Add small quantities of water to the bottom of the pot and add olive oil. Heat and add beef, tomato, ointment, red pepper, and garlic thoroughly. Steam sauce until brown beef and tender onion. Add powder, tamari, and water to curry. Cover tightly and cook for 30 minutes at a medium-low level, adding water when necessary.

Grilled Venison

- Four steaks of poison (every 4 ounces)
- Two cubic tablespoons of chopped rosemary
- Two spooky cubicle garlic
- Two cubicles fresh or dried thyme chopped
- 1/4 of a cup of extra virgin olive oil
- One cubicle tamari Pumper for flavor.

Marinate venison in the refrigerator for 4 hours, sealed. Remove the excess oil from the marinade. Place venison on the grill indoor or outdoor. Season with pepper and marinade brush. Cook once for 5-9 minutes, depending on the thickness and heat of the restaurant. For maximum juiciness and tenderness, serve medium to medium-rare.

Herb and Garlic Beef and Lamb

- Two cutting or lamb shoulder

- One tablespoon of minced garlic

- 1/2 teapot of dried rosemary

- 1/2 teapot of dried tarragon

- Two tablespoons lemon juice

- 1/2 teaspoon tamari pepper to taste

Position chops in baking dishes. Combine the remaining ingredients, pour over the chops, and then cook at 350 ° F. Till done (about 35-45 minutes).

Herbed London broil

- London broiled beef (1/2 lbs.) fat and sliced into four

- One tablespoon extra-virgin olive oil

- Two cloves of goose garlic, chopped

- Four tablespoons Salt-Free All-Free Seasoning*

Brush all sides with olive oil, garlic, and all-purpose sauce without seasoning. If you have time, let it last for up to an hour. Prepare a barbecue or grill preheat. Grill on each side between 8-10 minutes, depending on the thickness and choice for your beef. When broiled, cook meat two inches from heat to ideal condition (four minutes per side for rare).

Italian breaded steak

- 1/2 kg of lean, 1/2 cup of thin beef bread, 1/4 cup of tomatoes

- 1 cup of chopped tomatoes

- One small ointment, sliced

- One clove garlic, sliced

- One big, green bell pepper, cut into strips

- One zucchini,

Cut out into streaks of season meat. Humidify the bottom of a pan and add butter. Then add meat and brown on the sides, and drain any fat away. Fill the meat with broth, tomatoes, onion, and garlic. Cover and cook until meat is tender around 1 hour. Add green pepper, then courgettes, and remove another 5 minutes to cook.

Liver and Onions

- 4-6 ounces' free beef liver varie

- One tablespoon citrus fruit

- One tablespoon of pure water

- One tablespoon of pure olive oil

- One clove of garlic, 1-2 small onions

- Two tablespoons of tamari

Position the liver in the plate and rinse off with lemon fruit juice. Let the rest of the recipe stand while preparing.

Heat over low heat a covered sauté pot. Add water when hot, add olive oil, garlic, onions, and tamari. Steam-sauté until the onions appear to become translucent. Attach the liver to the pan and cook on each side for 3 minutes. Then cover the pot tightly and allow the liver to steam for 5-10 minutes, or until fully cooked, depending on the liver thickness. Remove the liver and coat it with the onion blend.

Marinated flank steak

- 1-1/2-pound steak flank

- A marinade of meat*

Clean and rinse steak flank. Place in a large lock bag with zipping. Remove marinade of beef. If you can, refrigerate for 1-4 hours. Better yet, let the steak marinate in the refrigerator overnight. Turn the bag from time to time to ensure that all aspects of the beef are marinade.

Set the oven rack to the correct level of grilling. Switch the oven to "broil." Put meat in the broiler pan. Brush with marinade and broil on one side for about 9 minutes. Remove, turn over the meat, and grill on the other side with the marinade, and return to the broiler for 8 minutes.

Remove meat and let it sit for 3 minutes or so. Slice thinly on the diagonal.

Marinated Pork Loin

- 1-1/2 pounds of pork separated

- Pork Loin Marinade*

Pork Pat dry. Place in a big zip lock bag. Add faraway pork marinade. Cool and marinate 1-4 hours, or overnight if you have time. Change the bag regularly to ensure each part of the meat gets some marinade. Bake in a meat thermometer for 1-1/2 to 2 hours until 185 ° F.

Water fireplace at 325 ° F. In a roasting pan, place pork and pour over the marinade. When needed, season pork with salt and pepper.

Take the pork from the bakery and put it on the cutting board. Enable 10 minutes to cool, then slice.

Cup Cube Steak with Wine

- Four wide open range Beef Cube steak

- 1/2 tablespoon red wine

- 12 ounces' fresh champignons, sliced

- Four cloves garlic, sliced

- Four tablespoon onion, sliced

- Two tablespoon butter Place the steaks of beef and marinate for at least 1 hour (better marinated overnight). Place wine, wine, and mushrooms in covered containers, garlic, onion, and parsley.

Cut marinade steaks and conserve marinade. Heat skillet and melt butter over medium heat. Add steaks, two at a time, except for a large pot. Braise steaks on each side for 2 to 3 minutes. Remove from skillet and place steaks on a shallow casserole or serving platter in one plate.

Add reserved marinade and heat before boiling, blend together meat juices. Cook to minimize liquid for a few minutes. Pour over steaks and serve as soon as possible.

Rabbit Stew

- Two extra virgin tablespoons of olive oil

- One rabbit (about 2 pounds), sliced in servings

- One tablespoon black pepper (optional) 1 large onion, chopping

- Two cloves fresh garlic, chopping

- 2 cups of chicken or veggie bread, two large carrots, chopping

- Three tablespoons celery,

Chopped 10-12 button mushrooms, split one small carrot, chopped 1 liter Place the oil over low heat in a large, heavy pot. In a pan and brown the rabbit parts (about 5 to 7 minutes per side) add two tablespoons of water and then olive oil. Attach the tamari, and the pepper scatter. In a low baking pan, put the browned rabbit, carrots, celery, mushrooms, chopped tomatoes, and kohlrabi.

Then, add the onion to the saucepan and simmer 7 to 10 minutes for low heat to soften. Remove garlic and cook for another 2 minutes, stirring. Bring broth to a boil and clean the browned bits on the bottom of the pot. Reduce heat; add rosemary and parsley, and simmer for two more minutes. Pour the rabbit and the vegetables into the sauce. Bake 45 minutes. 45 minutes. Place rabbit parts on a serving dish and apply restful pan juices on top.

Venison Pot Roast

- Two tablespoons extra virgin olive oil 3 - 4-pound venison pot roast Black pepper to taste

- Two tablespoons tamari

- 4-6 medium tomatoes, chopped one medium onion, chopped

- 1 cup celery, chopped

- One tablespoon parsley, minced two teaspoons oregano

- Three cloves garlic, minced

- 1 cup vegetable or beef broth

Stir in olive oil and brown roast on all sides in a Dutch oven. Garnish with pepper and tamari. Combine the remaining ingredients and scatter over the roast. Cover and bake at 325 ° F for 3-4 hours.

Variation: Using free-range beef, or any large cut of meat from a big game animal if venison is not available.

Yakitori Beef

- One pound of beef sirloin free-range, tartar 1/2 cup ·

- Two tablespoons of 1 clove of garlic lemon juice, crushed

- 1/2 teaspoon ginger, ground

- One tablespoon of extra virgin olive oil

- Two granny onions,

Finely chopped tamari blend, lemon juice, garlic, ginger, butter, and onion in a food processor or mixer and combine together. Place in a tray of wine. Thread meat on bamboo spreaders and marinade skewered meat, turn to cover every side. Cover and cool 4 hours; rinse. Arrange on the broiler pan and grill the heating element 5 to 8 inches. Freeze for 1/2 to 2 minutes; grill for 1 minute longer.

Seafood

Almond Crusted Snapper

- 1/2 teaspoon Salt-Free All-Purpose Seasoning*,

- Spike or 1/2 cup almonds, ground fine (or other nut or seed if you prefer)

- 1-pound red snapper

- half teaspoon black pepper (adjust to taste)

- Two tablespoons extra virgin olive oil Preheat oven to 350° F.

Rinse the fillets of fish and drive them dry. Add salt on both sides of the fish and pepper. Grind the almonds in a food processor to a finer powder, then run the device on brief explosions. Don't grind or sticky out the mixture.

In a glass baking dish, place one tablespoon of olive oil, then add water. Sprinkle with almond food and bake for 15-20 minutes or until the fish flakes with a fork easily. Eat lemon or lime.

Baked White Fish

- 1/4 cup raw macadamia nuts
- Two large tomatoes
- 1-pound halibut, turbot or other white fish
- One small onion, minced
- 1/4 teaspoon black pepper
- One egg white
- One tablespoon extra-virgin olive oil
- 1/2 teaspoon Salt-Free All-Purpose Seasoning*
- One medium onion, sliced
- One green bell pepper, chopped

Free All-purpose Seasoning (Salting Free) do not overwhelm or become sticky. Set aside. Set aside.

In a food processor or mixer, puree tomatoes. Set aside. Set aside.

In a food processor, chop the fish and the small onion. Remove the meal of the almond, pepper, and white egg. Mix well. Mix well. Cut 12 spheres.

In a baking dish, combine the oil, sliced onion, green pepper, and tomato purée. Arrange fish balls inside, cover, and bake for 40 to 45 minutes in 325 degrees F oven. Until serving, add the sauce.

Broiled Tilapia Pesto

- Four filets of tilapia (approx. 6 ounces each) 2 cloves of garlic, tough
- 1/3 cup fresh lemon juice one tablespoon of tamari

- One teaspoon of extra virgin olive oil two teaspoons of olive oiled Lemon slices

- Four tablespoons of Italian Basil Pesto*

Position fish on a flat plate. Toss together garlic, lemon juice, tamari, olive oil, and onion, and pour over fish. Marinate for 30 minutes or more.

On broiler pan, position the fish and grill with marinade. Broil 6 inches of heat, according to the thickness of the tilapia filets for 3 to 4 minutes. Place on each filet one tablespoon of Italian Basil Pesto out and take out the broiler pan. Turn the heat off the broiler and return the pot to the oven for 2 minutes to cook the pesto.

Serve with slices of lemon.

Cajun Filets

- 1/8 teaspoon garlic powder or one clove minced, fresh garlic

- Two tablespoons lemon juice one tablespoon tamari

- Two tablespoons olive oil

- catfish 1/8 teaspoon crushed red pepper or 2 to 1/2 pounds of fish filets - sole, trout, snapper

Coat all sides of the fish fillets with this combination. Preheat oven to 350 degrees F. In a shallow pot heats up lemon juice and tamari oil over low heat. Place the fillets side by side, overlapping slightly in a pot where necessary.

Mix together the dry spices and sprinkle over the fillets Bake for 20-25 minutes, based on filets size and fish condition (the longest catfish bakes). The pot -blacken, but that's all right; the liquid holds the fish moist. Serve immediately. Serve immediately.

- Four halibut fillets (4 ounces each)

- 1/4 cup fresh lime juice

- One tablespoon fresh lemon juice

- One teaspoon tamari

- Four green onions, sliced in 1/2 inch lengths one tomato, coarsely chopped

- One teaspoon chili powder

- chopped 1/2 cup red bell pepper

Place the halibut on a shallow baking platter. In a cup, mix lime juice, lemon juice, tamari, and chili powder and sprinkle over halibut. Marinate for 10 minutes, then transform once or twice.

Sprinkle over fish onions, peas, and peppers. Tent. Tent. Bake 30 minutes at 350 F or only until halibut flakes are in the center. Let stand for 4 minutes, sealed, before serving. Remove new cilantro to garnish.

Variation: You can use snapper, cod, or any other white fish if halibut is unavailable.

Dijonnaise Poached salmon

- 1/4 cup lemon juice

- Two bay leaves

- Four wild salmon filets (about 6 ounces each)

- One teaspoon Spike or 1/4 teaspoon salt

- 1/3 cup Omega 3 Mayonnaise*

- Two tablespoons Dijon mustard

Remove the citrus juice and the baking leaves and bring it to a boil. Reduce the heat to a frying bottle. For freshwater rinse trout, spray with spike and/or salt and drop the fish softly into the bowl. Cover and poach for nearly eight minutes.

Mix Omega 3 Mayonnaise and the Dijon mustard while the fish is poaching. When the fish is finished (must be opaque but still firm), remove the slotted spoon or spatula from the plate. Place over each filet onto the serving plate and spoon sauce.

Fish Filets in Red Sauce

- white wine1/2 cup dry or water

- One sprig fresh thyme (or 1/2 tablespoon dried)

- Two tablespoons extra virgin olive oil

- two medium onions, chopped

- Two cloves garlic, minced

- 2 cups fresh or canned tomatoes

- 1 cup black pitted olives

- 1/2 cup basil, chopped

- One sprig fresh rosemary (or 1/2 tablespoon dried)

- 1 or 1/2 pounds red snapper or other thick white fish, skinless

- Black pepper to taste (optional)

- regular salt to taste (optional)

- Morton Salt Substitute (optional)

Apply two spoonfuls of water to the deep skillet then olive oil. Remove the onion and simmer until soft. Spray with garlic and tomatoes. Raise heat, and allow some tomato juice to evaporate as you periodically stir. Add water or wine, and cook for another 5 minutes.

Stir in olives, basil part, rosemary, thyme, salt, and pepper. Cook flavors to mix for several minutes. Submerge fish in the sauce and cook for about 8 minutes over medium heat until the fish is clean and tender. Garnish with Basil dust.

Herbed Salmon

- Four wild salmon filets (about 6 ounces)
- One extra virgin olive oil
- Two cloves of garlic
- One teaspoon black pepper
- One teaspoon of caps
- 1 cup of pssol, chopped
- 1 cup of coriander, chopped
- 3 cup of lemon rind grated teaspoons
- 1 /2 cup of fresh lemon juice
- 1/2 teaspoon Spike or seasoning

Preheated oven at 350 ° F. Rinse and rinse the skin. Layer the baking sheet lightly oiled. Combine oil, garlic, spices, caps, pets, cilantro, lemon rind and juice and seasoning in a blender or food processor. Spread over fish. Spread over fish. Bake for 15 minutes or until the fish flakes with the fork are smooth.

Lemon Parslied Fish

- 1-pound whitefish or sole filets
- 1/4 cup lemon juice
- Two teaspoons extra virgin olive oil
- 1/4 teaspoon white pepper
- washed and minced 1/2 bunch fresh parsley (leaves only)
- One small onion, thinly sliced
- One small lemon washed well and thinly sliced

Cut the fish into serving-size portions. Remove the lemon juice and oil and sprinkle with seasoning. Arrange lemon and onion slices over the fish; sprinkle with the parsley. Cover for

5 minutes, and let stand. Bake for 15-20 minutes at 350 ° F, or quickly with a fork until the fish flakes.

Pecan Catfish

- 1/4 cup extra virgin olive oil

- 1/4 cup pecans, chopped fine

- One tablespoon lemon juice

- 1/4 teaspoon ground savory

- One teaspoon tamari

- 1/4 teaspoon red pepper flakes one teaspoon lemon rind, grated 2 pounds' catfish filets

Create pecan sauce by mixing 1/4 cup, less than one tablespoon of olive oil, pecans chopped, lemon juice, and salty. Mix well.

Combine tamari, lemon rind, and pepper flakes. Spread onto fish uniformly. Heat the skillet to non-stick over medium heat. Add one teaspoon of water and one cubit of olive oil. Brown filets over medium heat, turning once, until light brown.

Place the filets in 12x 8x two well-grated baking dish.

Drizzle lemon pecan sauce over filets. Once tested with a fork, bake uncovered at 350 ° F for 12 minutes or until the fish flakes easily.

Sardine Sushi

- Two tablespoons tamari

- Rice vinegar (optional)

- cucumber (1/2) cut into thin strips A few sprigs cilantro

- Several sheets of Nori (dried seaweed)

- 1/4 roasted red bell pepper, cut in thin strips

- 1/2 avocado cut into thin strips

- One can sardine, water-packed, a bit of ginger cut into small strips

Work at a time using one sheet of Nori seaweed. Place Nori sheet on a piece of plastic wrap or parchment. Starting approximately 1-1/2 inches from the edge of the sheet of seaweed, place ingredients (bell pepper, avocado, cucumber, cilantro, sardines, and ginger), form a line from top to bottom, running parallel to the edge of the sheet.

Sprinkle gently with the rice vinegar and tamari. Start rolling the ingredients from the edge nearest to you, tucking as you go so that it forms a smooth, tight roll. Wrap the rice, burrito-style, using the plastic wrap or parchment, and refrigerate for later use. It can be consumed as a roll or cut into thick discs and eaten as a snack or hors d'oeuvres.

Suggested Serving: 2 rolls

Note: When water-packed sardines are not provided, use oil-packed sardines. In this case, prior to use, pat the sardines dry with a paper towel.

3.3 Poultry & Eggs

Apricot Chicken

- Three free-range chicken breasts
- 1/2 pound mushrooms, cleaned and quartered
- 1 cup carrots, sliced
- One medium onion, chunked 1 cup celery, sliced
- Six medium apricots, fresh (dried OK if soaked for 3 hours first) Chicken broth to cover chicken pieces

Throw chicken bits into the crockpot beneath. Close to soup. Layer mushrooms, carrots, onions, celery, and apricots on top (do not cover them with broth, because there would be too much liquid). Cook for 6–7 hours at medium.

Baked Ginger Chicken

- 2-3 pounds' free-range chicken or chicken pieces
- Two tablespoons extra virgin olive oil
- Two tablespoons tamari
- Three tablespoons grated fresh ginger or
- One tablespoon ground ginger powder
- Two tablespoons grated fresh garlic or one teaspoon ground garlic powder

Clean the chicken and dry. Heat roasting pan with a spoonful of olive oil and put the chicken in an oiled oven.

Mix together the tamari with the second tablespoon of oil; add the ginger and garlic. Stir well and pour over the chicken, or brush on it. Bake 40-60 minutes (20 minutes per pound of bird), uncovered.

Cucumber Chicken (Delights)

- finely chopped 1/4 cup onion
- 1 cup cooked chicken breast, finely chopped three teaspoon Omega 3 Mayonnaise*
- Two tablespoons pecans, finely chopped
- 1-2 cucumbers, washed and peeled
- Salt-Free All-Purpose Seasoning*

Combine all components except the cucumber. Refrigerate for at least 2 hours, then cover. When ready to eat, slice the cucumbers into 1/4-inch thick slices. Chicken layer 1-2 teaspoons over rising cucumber

Crockpot Chicken

- Two carrots, sliced

- Two onions, sliced

- Two celery stalks with leaves, cut in 1-inch pieces

- 3-pound whole free-range chicken, skin and visible fat removed

- Two teaspoons tamari

- 1/4 teaspoon black pepper

- 1/2 cup chicken broth

- One teaspoon fresh or dried basil one teaspoon

Bring in the crockpot bottom carrots, onions, and celery. Stir in the chicken. Top with broth, herbs, and tamari. Sprinkle with basil on top. Cover and cook until cooked at low (8-10 hours). Use a spatula to cut chicken and vegetables.

Note: You can also use a high setting (chicken will be finished in 3 to 4 hours) on your crockpot, but you will need to raise the water to 1 cup.

Grilled Turkey

- 1-pound turkey breast cutlets (about 1/4" thick)

- Two tablespoons Dijon-style mustard

- One tablespoon Omega 3 Mayonnaise* Spike, black pepper and paprika to taste

- One teaspoon fresh lemon juice

- Two tablespoons chopped fresh parsley

Fill broiler with preheating. Coat broiler pan with a cooking spray, which is non-stick. If the non-stick spray is not available, rub some olive oil onto the bottom of the pan. Rinse on turkey and dry hold. In a small cup, add the mustard, mayonnaise, spike, and lemon juice.

Coat turkey one hand with half the mustard mixture. Broil for 5 minutes at around 4 inches from heat source. Turn and coat the turkey's other hand with the mustard mixture and sprinkle with pepper and paprika. Broil for 1 minute, or until browned on top. Cover with chopped parsley garnish.

Ostrich Burgers

- Two spoonsful of onion, finely sliced

- One clove of garlic, finely minced

- One spoonful of extra virgin olive oil

- 1 pound of soft veal meat

- one-fourth teaspoon of fresh ground black pepper

- One spoon of tea tamari

Clean onion and garlic in olive oil. Blend beef, tamari, and pepper in a thick mixture of onion and garlic. Cook in a pot: heat a pot over medium heat. Form 3 patties 1/2, "3-1/2," diameter, and sprinkle on each side for about two minutes. Grill: preheat the grill, brush the meat with oil, and grill for about four minutes, on either side. Serve grilled onions and/or sautéed mushrooms, guacamole, sliced tomatoes, and lettuce, if desired.

Poached Chicken

- 1/2 onion

- Two clove garlic, whole peeled

- One teaspoon tamari

- 4-5 whole pumice

- Two bay leaves

- One teaspoon dried rosemary

- One teaspoon

- One teaspoon dried thyme

- Two chicken breasts of free-range,

Skinless (about 4 ounces each) in the bottom of the frying pan, placed approximately 2 inches of water. Remove all vegetables, herbs, and seasonings and cook. Add chicken breasts, cover tightly, and cook for 15-20 minutes at medium-low heat, or until the chicken is done. With the slotted spoon, cover. Drink and serve hot or slice.

Variation: For poaching fish, this recipe can be altered by dropping rosemary, sages, and thyme and adding fresh dill or cilantro and savory season.

Poultry Cutlets

- 1/2 pounds' turkey or freestyle thighs
- 1 1/4 teaspoons spike
- Black chicken to taste
- One teaspoon of poultry
- One teaspoon butter
- 1/8 cup of lemon juice
- 1/8 cup of freestyles chicken or turkey stock with one 1/8-inch meat mallet.

Sprinkle with Spike, chicken, and black pepper. Place bowl or sprayed pan over medium heat.

In the bowl, melt butter and sear cutlets on both sides rapidly to brown (approximately 1 minute per side). Add lemon juice and simmer for 2 to 3 minutes more. Clear from the saucepan and heat the saucepan. Add stock and deglaze (residue of the pot stirring and loosening). Turn the heat up and reduce to half the air. Pour over poultry and serve as soon as possible.

Shitake Ostrich Steaks

- 2 pounds' ostrich steaks, 1/2-pound fresh shiitake mushrooms, one teacup of spike seasoning

- One tablespoon of freshly ground Black pepper

- Four tablespoons of virgin extra olive oil

- Three tablespoons of onion, fine chopped

- One cup of the beef stock Steam low steam non-stick skillet.

Remove one cubicle of water and two cubicles of olive oil.

Remove champagne and 1/2 tea cubicle tamari. Stir and cook until the champagne is lightly browned and tender (approximately 2-3 minutes). Set aside. Set aside.

Rinse the ostrich and rinse it dry. Sprinkle the salt and pepper gently on both ends. Heat a saucepan over medium heat, add two tablespoons of water and two tablespoons of olive oil Steam-sauté ostrich steaks on each side for 1 minute. Drop the winter, cover loosely to keep warm when preparing the sauce.

Add chopped onion. Pour off any remaining fat in the saucepan. Return to medium-high heat, then add beef stock. Cook quickly to say the sauce, around 1/4. Taking off power

Add medium mushrooms and medium. Add the ostrich to the bowl and cover it with the sauce. Sprinkle thyme chopped over autumn and serve.

Tarragon Turkey Patty

- 1/4-pound ground turkey

- Two tablespoons chopped onion

- One teaspoon fresh parsley, chopped to tablespoons macadamia nuts ground to a fine meal

- 1/2 teaspoon fresh thyme, chopped

- fine One teaspoon extra virgin olive oil

- 1/4 teaspoon dried tarragon

- One egg white

Mix all of the ingredients, except oil and nutmeal, in a small pot. Form the turkey mixture into a 3/4 "thick patty. Steam the skillet over medium heat, add water at a tablespoon, and then add oil.

Dredge the turkey patty in the nut meal, and put it in the skillet. Cook for around 5 minutes on either hand or while pricked with a fork, until the juices run loose. Don't let them overcook.

Turkish and Mushroom

- Two tablespoons extra virgin olive oil

- 1/4 pound of turkey

- 10-12 button mushrooms, grossly sliced

- Two stalks celery, grossly sliced

- 1-2 cloves of garlic, chopped thin

- One ointment, coarsely cut

- One tablespoon of fine grass* Tamari, to taste

Heat the pot and add a small amount of water. Then add oil and ground turkey, champagne, celery, garlic, onion, and fine herbs. Steam-fry before the turkey has been fried. Fill in the tamari to taste. If necessary, adjust the seasonings.

Variation: In this recipe, you can replace or add any remaining vegetables.

Turkey Breast Crockpot

- Two carrots, cut into one "lengths, three celery stalks, sliced

- Two onions, cut into three chunks of garlic, cut in 1 cup of chicken bread

- One bay leaf

- A few whole pepper grains

One teaspoon of poultry seasoned two tamari teacups Combine crockpot ingredients, coat, and cook at low temperatures for 5-8 hours.

Turkey Burger

- 1/4 pound of Turkish soil
- One clove of garlic, finely chopped one egg
- One teaspoon of tamari
- One teaspoon of onion

Two teaspoons extra virgin olive oil Mix together the whole ingredients with the exception of olive oil and form into a patty. Steam the medium-heat kettle, add two teaspoons of water, then oil. Add the patty and sauté steam for 8-10 minutes or until it's fried.

Turkey Meat Loaf

- 1/4 cup walnuts, ground fine
- 2 pounds ground turkey
- 1/2 onion, diced
- One zucchini, diced
- Eight mushrooms, chopped
- One medium carrot, grated
- A handful of spinach chopped fine
- One egg, well beaten
- Two teaspoons Spike

Grind walnuts in a blender but do not over-grind or they will get oily. Mix all ingredients together. Pat into a long loaf in a nine x13 pan. Bake at 350° F. for 90 minutes.

Turkish Stained Stage

- 2 pounds of beef, skinless

- One medium onion

- Two stalks of celery, chopped · one medium of tomatoes, chopped

- One medium of carrot, chopped

- 1/2 green of bell pepper, chopped (optional)

- Two cloves of garlic, chopped of fine

- One teaspoon of the spike, or seasoning

- One teaspoon of thyme

- One tablespoon of marjoram

- 2 cups of chicken stock

Place all ingredients in the crockpot and cook on low for 6 - 8 hours.

Eggs

Deviled Eggs

- 1/2 teaspoon Spike Black pepper to taste

- 1/4 teaspoon dill (optional) Paprika (optional)

- Six large organic eggs

- 1/3 cup Omega 3 Mayonnaise* 2 teaspoons Dijon mustard

Bring the water up over high heat to a boil. With a spoon, slowly slide eggs into the water and raising heat to simmer cook for 5 or 6 minutes. Pour hot water off and fill the saucepan with cold water to cool eggs instantly.

When the eggs are soft, peel them, and cut them lengthwise in half. In a small cup, scoop out the yolks and put whites on a serving platter. Stir in mayonnaise, mustard, and seasonings to the yolks.

Mash and mix well until soft. Fill the cavity with yolk mixture of every egg white half and sprinkle on top with dill or paprika.

Frittata

- 1/4 teaspoon black pepper four eggs
- One tablespoon olive oil
- 1/2 pound mushrooms, sliced
- One clove garlic, minced (optional)
- 1/2 cup onion, chopped
- 1/2 red bell pepper, chopped fine1/2 teaspoon Dijon mustard
- 2 cups vegetables, chopped (can use asparagus, broccoli, zucchini, spinach or greens) 1/2 tablespoon marjoram
- 1/2 teaspoon oregano
- 1/2 teaspoons Spike
- 1/8 cup parsley, chopped

Attach a large skillet with olive oil and switch heat to medium-low. Add onions, mushrooms, and garlic. Sauté until the onions are clear and smooth. Add chilies, herbs, and seasonings. Remove well and cook until vegetables turn bright green.

Break the eggs and pour the mustard into a pot. Mix well together and sprinkle in a skillet over vegetable mixture. Cook for about 4 minutes, until eggs are set. Serve with shredded parsley.

Huevos Rancheros

- 1 tablespoon couchette extra virgin olive oil
- 4-5 tomatoes, chopped
- 1/4 onions, cut

- Three garlic cloves squeezed through the press of the garlic or chopped Serrano or some other chili pepper to taste. Chili punch (optional)

- Four eggs

- Six large lettuce leaves

Set small saucepan to medium heat. Add two water teaspoons and then one oil tablespoon. Add tomatoes, onion, garlic, peppers, and powdered chili. Bring sauce to a boil, may heat and cook for approximately 10 minutes.

Brush with olive oil the bottom of the larger saucepan. Fry eggs gently "sunny side up." (Don't cook or overcook eggs on the top side).

Set out three leaves of lettuce on two plates each. Put two eggs on every leaf table. Cover the eggs with the other pan's sauce. The sauce cooks the tops of the eggs in half.

Spinach and Eggs

- One hard-cooked egg

- 2-3 cups of fresh spinach or mixed greens one small onion, chopped

- Salt-free All-Purpose Seasoning* or Spike for slice egg and greenery.

Slice egg and place over greens. Season to taste

3.4 Salads & Vegetables

Apple Turkey Salad

- 2 cups unpeeled apples, diced

- 1 to 1/2 teaspoons lemon juice

- 2 1/2 cups cooked organic turkey, diced

- 1 cup celery, diced

- 3/4 teaspoon Spike, or Salt-Free All-Purpose Seasoning*

- 1/4 teaspoon pepper (optional)

- Three tablespoons Omega 3 Mayonnaise*

Apples blend gently with lemon juice. Add leftover ingredients and toss gently. Serve on a lettuce plate or other plants.

Asian Salad

- One large head Bibb lettuce

- One large head Boston lettuce

- 2 stalks Chinese cabbage

- 1 cup bean sprouts

- 3/4 cup jicama, thin 1" strips

- 3 - 4 tablespoons Asian Dressing*

Pat lettuce and cabbage dry, tear into bite-size pieces, and put into a wooden salad bowl. Rinse bean sprouts and pat dry. Add sprouts and jicama. Dress with Asian Dressing. Toss lightly until all ingredients are coated.

Avocado Citrus Salad

- One orange, cut into chunks

- 1/2 pink grapefruit, cut into chunks

- 1/2 avocado, sliced thin

- Pine nuts (optional)

Combine. Sprinkle lightly with pine nuts, if desired. Add rice vinegar to taste.

Bean Sprout Salad

- 4 ounces' fresh bean sprouts

- One fresh green chili, seeded and sliced

- One small onion, finely sliced

- One teaspoon tamari

- One tablespoon lemon juice

Wash bean sprouts thoroughly and drain well. Mix all ingredients together. Refrigerate for several hours before serving.

Cabbage and Cherry Salad

- 2 cups cabbage, shredded

- One orange, peeled and chopped

- 1/2 cup jicama, peeled and chopped

- one cup pitted fresh or frozen sweet cherries

- 1/2 cup butter lettuce, washed, dried and torn into bite-size pieces

- 1/2 cup walnuts

Combine ingredients in a salad bowl and top with Ginger Dressing*. Serve cold.

Chicken and Grape Salad

- Romaine lettuce leaves, torn into bite-size pieces

- One head Belgian endive

- 1-1/2 cup cooked, chilled julienne slices of chicken breast

- 2/3 cup green or red seedless grapes

- Three tablespoons chopped walnuts Alfalfa sprouts as garnish

To assemble the salad, line a large serving platter or individual plates with romaine leaves. Quarter the Belgium endive and arrange Belgian endive, chicken pieces, grapes, and nuts on leaves.

Garnish with alfalfa sprouts if desired. Drizzle with 1-2 tablespoons of dressing per serving.

Chicken Salad

- 1/4 - 1/2 cooked chicken breast, sliced or diced
- 1-2 cups premixed salad greens
- One stalk celery, chopped
- One green onion, chopped Olive-Lemon Dressing*
- 2-3 tablespoons raw sunflower seeds or raw cashews

Mix all ingredients into a bowl, except seeds/nuts. Add the small-moderate amount of dressing and toss. Garnish with seeds/nuts.

Chopped Salad

- Coarsely chop the following vegetables in any combination: Carrots
- Cauliflower Broccoli Celery Cucumber Jicama Scallions Cabbage

Store in a covered container. Serve with Vinaigrette dressing* or lemon juice.

Confetti Salad

Eight cups of all kinds of mixed greens (for instance, spinach, red salad, green salad, roman, wild greens, cabbages, arugula, radicchio, kale, chard, etc.). Carefully wash, dry, and cut.

Chop and add all the following:

- Alfalfa sprouts Asparagus (rough) Bean sprouts
- Bell peppers (green, red, yellow) Carrots (no more than a carrot) Cucumber
- Herbs (dills, parsley, thyme, cilantro) Cohlrabi
- Owns (red, white, yellow or green) Pea pods (editable)
- Cups of radishes

- Summer pan, yellow and crookneck, mix with each other and all of the following

Egg-Shrimp Salad

- 2 cups pre-washed spinach
- 2-3 teaspoons flaxseed, freshly ground (use another seed or nut if you wish)
- 1-2 hardboiled eggs, sliced
- Three precooked shrimp, tails removed
- One tablespoon Mexican Guacamole*
- Two tablespoons of your favorite salsa

Spread spinach on a plate, sprinkle ground flaxseed, and arrange hardboiled egg slices on top. Add shrimp and top with Mexican Guacamole* and your choice of salsa.

Fennel, orange, and arugula Salad

- 1/2 cup shallots minced
- Three tablespoons extra virgin olive oil 1
- 1/2 tablespoons fresh lemon juice Spike seasoning
- Tamari flavor Black pepper
- Two major oranges peeled and sliced
- 7 cups of arugula, chopped
- One broad fennel bulb, cored, sliced
- One small red ointment, thinly slitted

Top with spike or tamari and pepper to taste. In a large bowl, combine arugula, fennel, and onion. Toss to the coat with sufficient dressing.

Hawaiian Chicken Salad

- four ounces red onion, cut into small pieces

- 1/2 cup raw macadamia nuts, chopped

- one pound grilled chicken breasts, sliced into thin strips

- eight ounces fresh green beans, blanched

- 8 ounces' yellow bell peppers, sliced into thin strips

- 8 ounces' cucumber slices

- 8 ounces' fresh papaya, cut into small pieces

- One teaspoon tamari

- 1/4 teaspoon ground black pepper (optional)

- 3/4 cup vinaigrette salad dressing

- 1/2 cup carrots, peeled, sliced into one thin strip

- eight ounces red bell peppers, sliced into thin strips

- one pound mesclun lettuce mix or other chopped salad greens

2-3 green onions, cut into 1 "thin strips in a wide mixing bowl, put lettuce/salad mixture, chicken, bell peppers, green beans, cucumber, red onion, and papaya. Season with tamari and pepper.

Drizzle the salad ingredients over the vinaigrette dressing and gently mix them together.

Sprinkle over each serving of the salad with the macadamia nuts. Garnish with green onions and sliced carrots.

Leftover Fish Salad

- 1-pound leftover fish and/or other seafood, already cooked

- Two medium tomatoes, coarsely chopped

- 1 cup celery, sliced into
- 1/2 inch slices 1/2 cup red onions, thinly sliced
- 1/4 cup fresh cilantro, chopped
- 1/2 cup fresh parsley, chopped
- 1/4 teaspoons Spike or seasoning
- 1/4 teaspoons black pepper
- Break fish/seafood into small chunks. In a large serving bowl, add all vegetable ingredients. Toss with Lemon Mint Dressing*. Add fish/seafood and toss in the salad.

Mediterranean Salad

- Two medium cucumbers, peeled and diced
- 3/4 cup tomatoes, chopped fine
- 3/4 cup celery, diced
- 1 cup Jerusalem artichokes (sunchokes), chopped fine
- 2 cups curly parsley, chopped
- 2 cups flat-leaf Italian parsley, chopped
- 1 cup fresh mint leaves, chopped
- One tablespoon pine nuts
- Three tablespoons fresh lemon juice
- Three tablespoons extra virgin olive oil, 1/4 teaspoon freshly ground black pepper (optional)
- One teaspoon Morton Salt Substitute or
- 1/2 teaspoon regular salt

Combine all chopped vegetables in a large bowl. Blend together the lemon juice, olive oil, salt, and pepper. Pour over the ingredients, and thoroughly flip. Four plates.

Raw Veggie Delight

- One zucchini, shredded
- One carrot, shredded
- 3-4 lettuce leaves, shredded
- A handful of alfalfa sprouts or bean sprouts
- A handful of cauliflower, chopped into small bite-sized pieces
- 1/2 red bell pepper, diced

A handful of red cabbage, chopped Shred zucchini, and carrots in a food processor. Put all of the above ingredients in a large salad bowl and mix it together. Top with Veggie Topping (below) or choose one of our Sauces and Dressings recipes.

Veggie Topping 2 tomatoes

- One stalk celery
- Two small-medium carrots Juice of one lemon 1/2 cup soaked seeds, nuts, or avocado, depending on desired thickness and consistency Blend the above five ingredients in a blender. Pour mixture over salad and mix thoroughly.
- One serving

Salad Nicosia

- 1/2 pound green beans
- Two eggs, hard-boiled
- 6 cups assorted lettuces or other greens
- Two cans tuna (substitute fresh grilled if you have it)
- Three tomatoes, cut into wedges
- Six anchovies (optional)
- One teaspoon capers (optional)

- 3/4 cup olives, pitted

- Two tablespoons red wine vinegar

- 1/2 cup extra virgin olive oil

- Morton Salt Substitute or regular salt (optional) Black pepper (optional)

- One shallot, minced

One teaspoon Dijon mustard Steam green beans for 4 minutes. Drain, dump into ice water to set the color. Refrigerate until time to use. Boil eggs cool and refrigerate until ready to use. Arrange greens on a platter. Top with tuna, green beans, eggs, tomatoes, anchovies, capers, and olives. Mix in small bowl or blender the red wine vinegar, olive oil, shallot, Dijon mustard, and salt and pepper to taste.

Note: A number of these ingredients can be prepared in advance and stored in the refrigerator until you are ready to assemble the salad. Improvise with the ingredients if you don't have certain things on hand.

Salmon Salad

- Four cups romaine lettuce leaves, torn into bite-size pieces

- 1 cup Jerusalem artichokes, peeled and cut into matchsticks

- 3/4 cup jicama, peeled and cut into matchsticks

- 8 ounces' sunflower sprouts (or any other sprouts you have)

- 1/2 avocado, cubed

- Two teaspoons capers (optional)

- 4-6 ounces' leftover baked or poached wild salmon, chunked 8-10 black or green olives, pitted

- Lemon wedges

- Three tablespoons Omega 3 Mayonnaise*

- One green onion, minced fine

- One teaspoon fresh parsley, chopped

- One teaspoon Dijon mustard

- One teaspoon fresh lemon juice

Arrange Romaine lettuce on serving platter. Arrange vegetables on top of lettuce. Top with salmon chunks and garnish with olives and lemon wedges. Mix mayonnaise, green onion, parsley, mustard, and lemon juice together. Serve as topping on a salad.

Shoestring Carrot Salad

- 3 - 4 large carrots, cut into shoestrings

- 1/2 medium onion, chopped fine

- 1/2 green bell pepper, chopped fine

- 1/2 teaspoon celery seed or

- 1-2 tablespoons chopped fresh celery

- 1/2 teaspoon dried parsley flakes or

- 1/2 tablespoon fresh parsley

- 1/2 teaspoon Salt-Free All-Purpose Seasoning*

- Black pepper to taste

- Two tablespoons extra virgin olive oil

- 1/4 cup lemon juice

Place carrots, onion, and green pepper in a steamer for 3-4 minutes only. Remove and place in a bowl. Add celery seed and parsley. Combine the seasoning, pepper, olive oil, and lemon juice. Pour over vegetables and blend the entire mixture well.

Spinach and Pink Grapefruit Salad

- 8 cups spinach (about 1/2 pound), washed, stemmed, chopped or torn into bite-size pieces two pink grapefruit, sectioned

- Grapefruit Vinaigrette*

Place spinach in a salad bowl with grapefruit sections and dressing. Toss well.

Spinach Salad

- Two bunches fresh spinach washed and stemmed

- One bunch scallions, chopped

- Two tablespoons lemon juice

- Two teaspoons tamari

- One tablespoon extra-virgin olive oil Black pepper to taste (optional)

Drain spinach, pat dry, and chop. Add scallions, lemon juice, tamari, olive oil, and pepper.

Variation: For some added heartiness, add either 1/4 cup chopped walnuts or one sliced hardboiled egg

Turkey and Broiled Eggplant Salad

- 1-pound eggplant

- 1-2 teaspoons tamari

- 1-2 teaspoons Salt-Free All-Purpose Seasoning*

- Two large heads of lettuce (leafy)

- Two cucumbers, shredded

- 1 cup cooked turkey, chunked

- One tablespoon capers (optional)

- 1/2 cup Olive Lemon Dressing*

Slice eggplant into slices about 1/4-inch-thick and sprinkle with tamari and Salt- Free All-Purpose Seasoning*. Broil eggplant until brown (about 3 - 4 minutes on each side).

While eggplant is broiling, tear washed lettuce into bite-size pieces and shred cucumbers. Plate the salads. Remove eggplant from broiler.

Cut turkey into chunks and divide over salads. Slice cooled eggplant and arrange over salads. Garnish with capers and drizzle with Olive Lemon Dressing*.

Turkey Citrus Salad

- 2 cups turkey, cooked and chopped

- 1/2 cups celery, chopped fine

- 1/4 teaspoon Salt-Free All-Purpose Seasoning*

- 1/4 teaspoon curry powder

- One orange

- 1/2 cup seedless grapes

- Two tablespoons Omega mayonnaise*

Combine turkey, celery, and seasonings in a bowl. Peel and chop the orange. Add orange, grapes, and mayonnaise. Toss gently to mix.

Warm Beef and Walnut Salad

- Assorted lettuce leaves, torn into pieces

- 8 ounces' lean beef strips (or buy a thick piece of fillet or rib-eye steak and slice thinly) 1/4 cup red pepper (any kind), cut into thin strips

- One small onion, cut into wedges

- Two teaspoons extra virgin olive oil one tablespoon walnut pieces Walnut dressing (see below)

- One tablespoon fresh chives, chopped

Walnut dressing

- 2-3 teaspoons walnut oil or extra virgin olive oil
- Two teaspoons white wine vinegar
- One teaspoon Dijon mustard Black pepper (optional)

Warm Nut and Cress Salad

- One tablespoon extra-virgin olive oil
- One large garlic clove
- Two tablespoons pine nuts
- Two tablespoons hazelnuts, finely chopped
- 1/2 teaspoon tamari
- 1/4 teaspoon black pepper (optional)
- 1-pound watercress washed and finely chopped

Cut the garlic clove lengthwise in half, then add to the oil. Cook on for 2 minutes, continuously stirring. Cut the garlic, and throw away.

Add all nuts and cook for 5 minutes or until they are slightly browned. Add tamari and pepper Cook 2 to 3 more minutes.

Working fast, toss watercress into nut and seasoning mixture, making sure it is well coated and barely heated through. If left too long, it loses some of its crispiness. Serve immediately.

Wild Greens Salad

- 6 cup mixed wild greens (whatever you can have in your area)
- Four teaspoons of fresh citrus juice
- Four teaspoons of tamari walnut
- One teaspoon of tamari
- 1-2 teaspoons of capers (optional) Whisk in oil slowly.

Spray with tamari or any other flavor. Pour over the greens and toss until dressed evenly. Garnish with capers. With capers. Serve at once. Serve at once.

Note: Wild greens in your region may include: chickweed leaves, salmon miners, lamb's salads, dandelion greens, wild mustard, purslane, lamb's quarters. If there are no wild greens available, look for rare greens locally available in certain supermarkets, health food stores, ethnic markets, or local farmers ' markets.

Vegetables

Apples 'n Onions

- Two tablespoons olive oil

- Four large Spanish onions, sliced

- Three large cooking apples, sliced

- 1/2 cup water or free-range chicken stock

- Two teaspoons tamari

- Dash of nutmeg

Preheat non-stick skillet. Moisten the bottom of the skillet with a little water, then add oil. Add onion slices and cook until nearly soft. Add sliced apples and 1/2 cup water or chicken stock. Cover and cook for 15 minutes, or until tender but not mushy apples. Sprinkle with and drink with nutmeg.

Baked Cabbage with Dill

- Cotton with 1/4 cup of water

- 1 cup of finely sliced cabbage

- Two teaspoons dried or two fresh dill tablespoons, fine chopped

Three tablespoons of olive oil preheating the oven to 350 ° F. Place the bottom of the baking dish with water. Remove chops in slices. Sprinkle with chopped dulse and dill, drizzle with olive oil. Olive oil. Cover with foil tightly and cook for 35 minutes or until col is tender.

Braised Onions, Shallots and Leeks

- One teaspoon extra virgin olive oil

- Three red onions, cut into thick wedges

- 3 Vidalia (or yellow) onions, cut into thick wedges 4 or 5 shallots, halved

- Three leeks, cut lengthwise, rinsed well and sliced into 2" lengths Fresh basil, minced, or dried basil

- juice of 1 lime

Heat deep skillet over low heat. Moisten the bottom of the skillet with one teaspoon water and then add oil.

Add onions and cook until they begin to soften (about 10 minutes), stirring occasionally. Add shallots, stir and cook, 4 - 5 minutes. Stir in leeks and continue cooking until they are bright green and tender (about 5 minutes). Add a little more water and a sprinkling of basil. Cover and simmer until any remaining liquid has been absorbed. Stir in lime juice and remove from oil.

Broccoli with Garlic and Lemon

- One bunch broccoli, about 1 pound

- 1/4 cup extra virgin olive oil

- Three cloves garlic, cut into thin slivers

- 1/8 teaspoon pepper

- Three tablespoons fresh lemon juice

Cook broccoli in a large saucepan of boiling water 5-6 minutes, or until tender-crisp. Drain in a colander. Arrange on a serving dish and cover to keep warm.

In a small frying pan, warm olive oil over low heat. Stir in garlic and cook slowly until golden brown, being careful not to burn the garlic (about 1-2 minutes). Add pepper and lemon juice. Pour sauce mixture over broccoli.

CABBAGE ROLL-UPS

- Chopped shrimp

- Avocado, sliced into thin strips (small to moderate amount) Cucumber, sliced into thin strips

- Roasted red pepper, sliced into thin strips Roasted zucchini, sliced into thin strips Chopped cilantro or parsley

- Sesame seeds (small amount) Leftover vegetables Steamed, cold green beans

- Roasted or raw onion, chopped Green onion sliced into thin strips Minced garlic

- Chopped fresh tomato

Use several leaves of green cabbage. Steam them for a couple of minutes just to soften. Remove from steamer and allow to cool. Fill with any combination of the above ingredients.

Mushrooms with Cauliflower

- green onions 1/3 cup (with tops), thinly sliced

- one cup chicken broth

- One large head of cauliflower

- One teaspoon extra virgin olive oil

- 1/4 pound fresh mushrooms, thinly sliced

Boil over medium heat, continuously stirring cook and stir for 2 minutes. Place the cauliflower in a wide bowl; pour over the mushroom mixture, and serve immediately. Steam the whole cauliflower until tender (about 20 minutes) in a saucepan containing 1 inch of water. Meanwhile, medium heat oil mushrooms and onions until mushrooms in a skillet are tender. Remove the chicken's broth.

Celery Slaw

- One big bunch of celery, cut fine

- Two red bells of pepper, cut fine

- 3 or 4 tomatoes

- 4 ounces of fresh walnuts

 Place celery and peppers in one cup. In a blender, cover and mix the tomatoes and walnuts until smooth. Garnish with celery and peppers.

Cole Slaw

- One colt, very thinly sliced

- One tiny medium carrot, shredded

- 1/2 white or red onion, slenderly

- One small, soft, green apple, shredded (optionally)

- One teaspoon Spike seasoning

- 1/2 teaspoon freshly ground black pepper

- 1/4 cup rice vinegar

Mix together seasonings, vinegar, and oil and pour over vegetables. Toss very well. Toss very well. Cover and cook for a total of 1 hour before serving.

Note: With this recipe, you can use all green chops, half-red chops, or a combination of black, red, Napa, or curly chips. The total amount of chalk should equal one full head of chalk or approximately 2-3 pounds.

Variations: Remove the rice vinegar and add 1/2 cup vinegar. Mix the vinegar with Dijon mustard 1/2 Tablespoon. Sprinkle one tablespoon full of caraway seed in a slaw. Cut the apple and sprinkle with three tablespoons of fresh dill chopped or two tablespoons of dried dill.

Remove rice vinegar from the dressing and add by two teaspoons of Omega 3 Mayonnaise* and one garlic clove blended with the cider vinegar. Pour over the salad and mix thoroughly.

Cooked Cabbage

- One small head of chalk

- One extra virgin teaspoon of olive oil

- 1/2 teaspoon of cool Homeric (or 1/4 teaspoon of dried)

- 1/2 teaspoon of fresh oregano (or 1/4 teaspoon of cooked oregano)

- 1/2 teaspoon of fresh thyme (or 1/4 teaspoon of chalk-dried)

Moisten with one tablespoon of water, apply one tablespoon of olive oil and heat at medium-low. Add chicken and blend, rosemary, oregano, and thyme.

Turn the heat to low, cover, and stir every few minutes to avoid burning. Cook for seven to ten minutes.

Variation: Instead of the spices mentioned above, using ginger and garlic as flavorings. If fresh ginger and fresh garlic are used, add about 5 minutes to the cooking.

Leeky Carrots

- One tablespoon extra-virgin olive oil

- Four tablespoons free-range chicken stock

- Three medium leeks, white and palest green parts only, rinsed and chopped

- Four large carrots, peeled and sliced

- Pinch of nutmeg (optional)

- Salt-Free All Purpose Seasoning (to taste)

Salt-free all-in - a-use seasoning (for taste) Remove the leeks and carrots, cover, and cook for around 8-10 minutes over medium-low heat or until tender. Stir often until leeks and carrots start to turn golden. Uncover and sauté. Remove the musk, if necessary. Serve and add seasoning.

Mashed Cauliflower

- One tablespoon of butter

- Two tablespoons olive oil

- 1/4 cup of water

- One clove of garlic (optional)

- Six cups cauliflower, chopped with fine ·

- Two tablespoons tamari

Onion powder to taste Add butter, olive oil or warmer, mix, toss in a large pot, oven, or electro-skillet (on the lowest temperature); stir. Cook on low heat until very soft cauliflower. Tamari and onion powder season.

With a hand blender or paste, the whip is smooth and crispy until the cauliflower. Use Gravy* with Mushroom.

Mustard Greens with Vinaigrette

- 2 cups of water

- 1/4 teaspoon tamari

- one-pound washed, mustard greens

- 1/4 inch strips Balsamic Vinaigrette* dressing

I am using a large skillet with a lid to add water and tamari and bring to a boil. Add the prepared vegetables, cover, and cook over high heat, occasionally stirring until tender for around 5 minutes. Drain in a colander, moving greens to the side using a cooking spoon to draw out excess moisture.

Ratatouille

- Two large onions, thinly sliced
- Two large eggplants sliced 1/2" thick
- Four ripe tomatoes stemmed and sliced thickly
- Four red or yellow bell peppers stemmed, seeded and sliced into
- 3-4 pieces
- Ten cloves garlic, peeled
- One teaspoon fresh rosemary or thyme
- One tablespoon tamari
- Black pepper to taste (optional)
- 1/2 cup extra-virgin olive oil
- Two tablespoons fresh parsley or basil, minced Preheat oven to 350° F.

Create a layer of the onion and then eggplant, tomatoes, peppers, garlic, basil, tamari, and pepper in a sealed casserole dish repeat layers where appropriate. Cover with olive oil and put it in the oven.

Bake in for about an hour. If the mixture is too warm, reveal another 15 minutes and bake again. If too warm, add a small amount of water or chicken stock and bake for another 15 minutes. Garnish with basil or parsley and serve.

Roasted Vegetables No. 1

- Four yellow summer squash

- Five zucchini
- Two red, yellow or orange peppers
- 15 - 20 small button mushrooms
- One red onion
- Three tablespoons extra virgin olive oil
- Three cloves garlic
- Two teaspoons tamari
- Dried cilantro or basil, chopped

Trim ends from summer squash. Cut into a roundabout 1/4" thick. Trim to zucchini ends. Cut into half, and then 3 or 4 bits. Break peppers into strips. Cut the onion into half, then wedges, leaving the root end in place so that the onion stays together during roasting.

Blend butter, garlic, and tamari together. In the mixture, throw vegetables. Spread about 15 minutes on the wide pan roast at 400 ° F. Sprinkle with basil or cilantro from the oven.

Note: Roasted vegetables can be made once a week for use as a snack or meal portion and stored in the refrigerator.

Roasted Vegetables No. 2

- Four medium carrots
- One eggplant, sliced about 1" thick
- two to four zucchini or summer squash halved 2-3 small onions, cut in quarters
- 1/4 cup extra virgin olive oil
- Three tablespoons fresh lemon juice

Connect olive oil and lemon juice to the vegetables Bake 35 minutes at 350 ° F with carrots and onion. Attach eggplant and zucchini and bake for another 20 minutes, turning if too brown.

Roasted Yellow Peppers

- Four large yellow bell peppers, about 2 pounds

- Three tablespoons extra virgin olive oil

- Two tablespoons shredded fresh basil, or

- 1 to 1/2 tablespoons chopped fresh parsley combined with

- One teaspoon dried basil Pepper to taste

Preheat oven to 475° F. Set peppers on a baking sheet. Brush with one tablespoon

Oil to lightly coat peppers.

Bake for 20 minutes, until the leaves start blistering (turning once or twice). Place the peppers in a brown bag or plastic bag for 10 minutes. Remove the pepper skins.

Take off roots, seeds, and membranes. Tear the peppers into four to six parts each. On a serving plate laid roasted peppers square. Sprinkle with parsley, basil, and new ground pepper.

Sautéed Broccoli Italian Style

- One head broccoli, cut into small flowerets, stems thinly sliced

- One teaspoon extra virgin olive oil

- 2 or 3 cloves garlic, minced

- One onion, diced

- four or five button mushrooms brushed clean and thinly sliced

- one or two tomatoes, diced

I am taking a wide pot of water to boil overheat. Remove broccoli and cook around 3 minutes until light green, but not fully tender. Plunge into cold water to stop the process of cooking and preserve the bright color.

Over medium heat, heat skillet. Moisten one teaspoon water in the base of the skillet, then add oil. Add garlic, onion, and champagne Cook for 2-3 minutes and stir. Add tomatoes and whisk thoroughly cover and cook for 10-15 minutes. Remove cover and incorporate broccoli. Simmer for 2-3 minutes, uncovered. Serve hot. Serve hot.

Spicy Wilted Greens

- Three teaspoons extra virgin olive oil

- Two tablespoons of shallots, hacked

- One teaspoon of ginger, ground

- Two teaspoons of ground pumpkins

- Two teaspoons of turmeric

- One teaspoon of coriander

- One teaspoon of jalapeno

- 1/2 squatting pound of tamari

- 1/2 teaspoon of tamari-1/2 pounds of chard (2 squats), thin sliced

- One squatting of scalp

- One squat of a teaspoon of ginger attaches the shallots, cumin, and ginger for 3 minutes. Stir frequently; do not encourage burning ingredients.

Add turmeric, jalapeno, tamari, and coriander. Three minutes longer, sauté. Remove greens and scallions and blend together with a mixture of oil and spice. Cover and encourage greens to wake, occasionally stirring. It takes about 10-12 minutes for collards; it takes about 8 minutes for chard. If too much liquid is present, remove the cover, turn the heat up and cook moisturizing greens. Serve immediately. Serve immediately.

Note: This recipe can be fired or simply flavored by changing the quantity of jalapeno.

Steamed Asparagus

- One bunch of fresh asparagus (green or white)

- One teaspoon of lemon juice

- One teaspoon of a fresh cat, minced

Put one inch of water with the steamer placed into the sealed pot to simmer. Wash asparagus and cut stiff ends steam up to the crunchy tender. Bring into a steamer. Serve with lemon juice and pomegranate.

Stir-Fried Bok Choy

- Two tablespoons extra virgin olive oil

- One large onion quartered and thinly sliced

- One medium-large bok choy (10-12 ounces), chopped crosswise in medium-large chunks one teaspoon grated fresh ginger, more or less to taste

- Two teaspoon tamari (optional)

Moisten a little water on the bottom of the stir-fry pan or big skillet, then add oil and heat. Attach onion, and sauté until golden over medium heat. Apply bok choy (stalks and leaves) and ginger to taste. Stir-fry quickly, before wilted leaves. Tamari season with.

Stuffed Mushrooms

- 1/3 cup pine nuts

- fresh basil, packed leaves, chopped 1/3 cup

- Three cloves garlic, minced

- packed leaves, fresh cilantro, chopped 1/3 cup

- One tablespoon lemon juice

- Two tablespoons tamari to taste

- One tablespoon extra-virgin olive oil

- one cup tomato, chopped

- eight-ten large button mushrooms

Place all ingredients, except for champignons and tomatoes, in a food processor and pulse chop several times. Stop rubbing the sides down and repeat. Continue to add tomatoes and pulse chop until you just blend. Maintain the mixture in a coarse form, more like a pesto than a purée. Spoon into mushroom caps and brush with olive oil Bake at 350 ° F for 10-15 minutes.

Tomato Cups

- Six small tomatoes

- 1/2 tiny cucumbers, chopping fine

- Two candy sticks, chopping green onions, chopping fine

- 1/2 cup of fresh parsley, chopped

- One tablespoon of fresh mint, minced

- One clove garlic, chopped 1/2 cup of pine sticks

- One tablespoon of lemon juice

- One tablespoon of tamari (optional) Add pulp to other ingredients (save some garnish with parsley) and blend well. Fill half of the tomato.

Tomatoes Dijon

- Four cloves of garlic, mashed

- One tablespoon of Dijon mustard

- 1/2 teaspoon of dry mustard All-properly sauced* and spicy (to be tasted)

- Two extra-virgin olive oil tablespoons

- Four small tomatoes, diced in half bowl, garlic, Dijon mustard, dry mustard, and savory.

Add oil, whisking until smooth, a little at a time. In the oiled baking dish, put tomatoes and spread the mustard mixture. Cook the tomatoes for 1 minute or until the tops are bubbling and golden.

Vegetables and Dip

- One middle carbonate

- One small jicama

- One red pepper, seeded

- Two medium squash

- Four medium squash

- 2 cups of flowers broccoli

- 2 cups of cauliflowers

One cup of snow or sugar snap peas Cut into sticks kohlrabi, jicama, pepper, squash, and celery. Break broccoli and cauliflower into tiny blooms. Tie the peas with snow if desired. Arrange to dip in the middle of the tray with a cup of Mock Sour Cream.

Vegetables in Ginger Sauce

- 1/2 tablespoons of broccoli oil

- 3 cups of chopped broccoli, sliced into quarter heads

- One head fennel washed in small pieces

- Two carrots, chopped

- 1 cup of fresh spinach, chopped

- Three cloves of garlic, chopped

- One tablespoon ginger, chopped

- 3 cups of fresh basil, cut

- One tamari teaspoon

- One red pepper
- One tablespoon of chopped basil.

Steam the medium-high non-stick skillet, and when dry, add two tablespoons of water to the pan and then add olive oil. Then add garlic, ginger, basil, chili, and scallions. Sauce, stirring well for one minute. Remove carrots and fennel and remove another minute of stirring. Remove broccoli and stock of chicken. Cover 30 seconds. Cover 30 seconds. Remove from heat and decorate with scallions.

Walnut Watercress Stir Fry

- Two teaspoons extra virgin olive oil

- One teaspoon of fresh ginger, skinned and rough

- A blanket of watercress, clogged

- 1/4 of a teaspoon of red potatoes

- One tablespoon of tamari

- Five tablespoons of chopped walnuts

- One teaspoon of walnut oil (optional)

Moistened bottom of wide skillet or wok with a limited quantity of water. Add olive oil. Include olive oil. Only after the oil is hot, stir in the ginger and cook for about 30 seconds until fragrant. Fall the cress, tamari, red pepper, and walnuts. Stir-fry until wilted but not overcooked, for about 3 minutes. Serve mild, chopped walnut oil, if desired.

Zucchini Sauté

- Two tablespoons water

- One large red onion, sliced thin

- Two small zucchinis, sliced into 1/4 inch rounds

- Two small yellow summer squash, sliced into 1/4 inch rounds one large ripe tomato, chunked

- One handful of fresh basil, chopped

Small pan with fire. Add two spoonsful of sugar, and then onion. 5 Seconds to drizzle. Attach the courgettes and the squash during the season. Only rock for about 5 minutes, occasionally. Garnish with Basil and Pepper. Cover and cook for another five minutes, or until everyone mixes.

3.5 Soups

Chicken Vegetable Soup

- Two cloves garlic

- One medium onion

- One tablespoon extra-virgin olive oil

- 2 quarts' low-salt chicken broth

- Two chicken breasts, bone, and skin removed

- Six tomatoes (or 24 ounces canned tomatoes if fresh not available)

- Two zucchinis, chopped

- 8 Brussels sprouts or other vegetables, chopped

- half cup fresh parsley

- half tablespoon turmeric Pinch of pepper (optional)

Sauté garlic and onion in a little olive oil in a soup pot. Add broth and bring to a boil. Add chicken. Simmer 30 minutes. Remove chicken, cool, and dice. Add vegetables and spices. Simmer another 15 - 20 minutes. Return chicken to the pot and serve when chicken is reheated.

Variation:

Substitute a turkey breast for the chicken.

Note:

Using the leftover soup for the next few days for breakfast, lunch, or dinner

Cilantro Chicken Broth

- 32 ounces' free-range organic chicken broth

- Two bunches of cilantro (leaves only), chopped fine

- One small minced onion (optional)

- 1/4 cup parsley, chopped

- One tablespoon tamari

Wash the coriander and the petroleum. Just finely cut the leaves of both. Chop it finely while using onion, as well. To the chicken broth, add all the chopped ingredients and tamari. Heat slowly until the hot broth and soft onion.

Curried Squash Soup

- One tablespoon extra-virgin olive oil

- 1 cup thinly sliced carrots

- 1/4 cup diced onion

- 1 cup zucchini, thinly sliced

- 1 cup yellow summer or patty pan squash, thinly sliced

- Two teaspoons chopped fresh parsley

- One teaspoon tamari 1/8 teaspoon pepper

- 1-2 teaspoons curry powder (to taste)

- 2 cups organic chicken broth

Cook onion in oil until translucent in one 1/2-quarter casserole. Remove all remaining ingredients except broth cover and cook over low heat, stirring periodically until the vegetables are tender. Remove the broth and cook. (Add more broth or some water if you want a thinner soup.)

Reduce heat to mild, and cook until vegetables are soft (about 20 minutes). Remove from heat and slightly allow to cool. Remove 2/3 of the soup from the pan and reserve; pour in the remaining soup into the blender and process until smooth at low speed. In a saucepan, blend pureed and reserved mixtures and reheat at low temperature, constantly stirring until dry.

Gazpacho

- 1 cup fresh tomato juice (see below)
- Four ripe tomatoes, quartered
- One small onion, coarsely chopped
- One clove garlic, peeled
- Two tablespoons lemon juice
- 1 - 2 tablespoons Spike
- half teaspoon cayenne pepper or hot chilies if you prefer
- One sprig fresh parsley
- Three scallions, chopped fine
- Two cucumbers, peeled and chopped

Make fresh tomato juice by adding multiple chunks of tomato to 1 cup of water in a blender and blend at a high pace.

In a blender or food processor, add all ingredients until the vegetables are well diced but NOT pureed. Serve with ice.

Italian Beef Soup

- 1-pound organic lean ground beef
- One tablespoon olive oil
- One small onion, chopped
- 1 cup chopped celery
- 1 cup chopped carrot

- One clove garlic, minced

- 1/8 teaspoon freshly ground pepper five medium tomatoes, diced

- Two medium tomatoes pureed 28 ounces' vegetable broth

- half cup fresh loosely chopped basil leaves

- One tablespoon chopped fresh thyme

- half (8-ounce) container sliced fresh mushrooms

Cook ground beef about 5 minutes or until golden, in a large Dutch oven; drain and set aside. Dutch oven heats the same over medium heat. Add two spoonsful of water and then add butter, onion, celery, carrot, and garlic. Drizzle for about 5 minutes or until vegetables are tender. Add chili pepper. Add onions, broth, basil, and thyme to taste.

Let simmer uncovered for 20 minutes over medium-low heat, stirring occasionally. Attach the mushrooms and beef and cook for another ten minutes.

Note: This is an extremely adaptable recipe. You should add your favorite veggies, and delete those you don't!

Louisiana Gumbo

- Three tablespoons extra-virgin olive oil

- 2 cups onion, chopped

- 1 cup celery, chopped

- Two large tomatoes, chopped

- 8 cups of organic chicken stock

- 8 cups pure water

- Four cloves garlic, minced

- Tamari, black pepper and red pepper

- 1/2 - 1-pound fish (any fish), in chunks

- 2 pounds' shrimp, peeled and deveined
- 1 cup frozen clams
- One tablespoon parsley, finely chopped
- 1/2 teaspoon "gumbo file" (dried, ground sassafras leaves)

Moisturize the bottom of the large soup kettle with two tablespoons of water, then add medium heat oil and heat until dry. Add onions and celery. Cook the onions until they are wilted, then add the tomatoes, chicken stock, water, and garlic.

Cook for a half-hour over medium heat and sprinkle on taste with tamari, black pepper, and red pepper. Assemble vegetables, shrimp, and clams cook ten more minutes. Sprinkle a splash of gumbo file on each gumbo platter served.

Minestrone

- One tablespoon extra-virgin olive oil
- Four cloves garlic, crushed
- One medium onion, chopped
- Three stalks celery, sliced
- One medium carrot, chopped
- One zucchini, chunked
- One tablespoon Italian seasoning
- One teaspoon Spike
- 1/2 teaspoon ground black pepper
- Two tomatoes, seeded and chopped
- 1-quart vegetable or free-range chicken stock
- 1 cup cabbage, shredded
- 1/2 cup Italian Basil Pesto*

Moisten with a bit of water the bottom of a soup pot or Dutch oven, then add the olive oil and heat. Add onions and garlic, and cook over medium heat until the onion is tender. Add celery, carrot, and zucchini to taste. Continue cooking for about 5 minutes, sometimes stirring.

Stir in seasonings, onions, stock, and bring to a boil. Reduce heat to a total of 10 minutes and simmer. Adjust of color, flavor, and seasonings.

Ladle into bowls and serve on top of each serving with one tablespoon of Italian Basil Pesto*.

Note: The longer this soup is simmering, the stronger it will get.

Scallion Soup

- Three teaspoons extra virgin olive oil

- 1 cup zucchini, shredded

- 1/2 cup white onion, chopped

- One clove garlic, minced

- one cup scallions, chopped

- 1/2 cup chives, chopped 2

- 1/2 cups chicken broth

- Two teaspoons tamari

Cook the courgettes, onion, and garlic in oil over low heat in a saucepan. Cook for about 5 minutes and stir occasionally. Add scallions and tablespoons of chives, minus two. Cook and serve until the scallions are ready, for about 2 minutes. Add broth and tamari and start to cook for another 2 minutes. Pretty cool.

Place the mixture in the blender and process to puree at low speed. Heat up and change the seasoning as necessary. Serve topped with chives left over.

Steak and Vegetable Soup

- 1-pound organic round steak
- One teaspoon dried basil or two teaspoons fresh basil, chopped
- 1/2 teaspoon Salt-Free All-Purpose Seasoning*
- 1/4 teaspoon pepper
- Two cloves garlic, crushed
- One tablespoon extra-virgin olive oil 32 ounces' organic beef stock
- two cups homemade Tomato Chili Salsa*
- one cup cabbage, chopped
- one cup zucchini, chopped
- 1/2 cup onion, chopped
- one cup celery, chopped
- one cup mushrooms, sliced
- 1/4 cup carrots, chopped
- one cup fresh spinach, torn into small pieces
- one cup fresh Swiss chard
- half cup fresh basil, cilantro or parsley (or all three), for garnish

Cut beef into 1/4-inch-thick strips; cut each strip into 1-inch pieces. In a medium bowl, combine beef, basil, seasoning, pepper, garlic, and oil; toss to coat.

Heat, over medium-high heat, a Dutch oven or large saucepan until dry. Apply two spoonful of water, then apply the beef mixture. Stir and cook for 4-5 minutes or until browned. With the exception of spinach and chard, pour in beef stock, salsa, and vegetables. Take to a boil over medium to high heat.

Reduce to low heat; simmer for ten minutes. Stir in chard and spinach. Garnish with fresh basil, parsley, or cilantro for any soup serving.

Note: Freezes well on this soup. Cool absolutely and placed in plastic bags or containers for freezer

3.6 Juices and Smoothies

Aloha Smoothie

- Two tablespoons flax seeds
- Two tablespoons raw macadamia nuts
- Two tablespoons raw almonds
- Two tablespoons pecans
- Two slices of organic ginger root one papaya
- About two cups of pure water Stevia to taste

Soak nuts and seeds, rinse overnight. Attach seeds, nuts, ginger, papaya, and some water to mix. Place the cap on top and blend until smooth. Add the remaining water at a time and continue to blend until all the water has been applied. Stir in stevia to try.

Apricot Apple Flaxseed Smoothie

Three fresh apricots pitted

- 1/2 medium apple, chunked
- Two tablespoons flax seeds
- 1/8 cup lemon juice
- one cup pure water Dash of cinnamon Stevia to taste

Soak the seeds of flax overnight, before using this recipe. Seeds drain. Place and process all ingredients in a blender or food processor until smooth, adding more water if needed.

Berry Nut Shake

- 3 cups pure water
- Two tablespoons almonds
- Two tablespoons pine nuts
- One tablespoon flax seeds
- 2/3 cup blueberries
- 1/4 teaspoon nutmeg Stevia
- 1/2 teaspoon vanilla

Soak the seeds of flax overnight, before using this recipe. In a food processor, process nuts on high until the bottom. Slowly add water and cycle. Stir in fruit, cinnamon, and nutmeg. Add stevia to taste, to sweeten. Mix well.

Notes: If you would like a cooler shake, cover some of the water with ice. This recipe can be varied by using any nuts or seeds you like.

Cucumber Mint Smoothie

- Two medium cucumbers, peeled
- Two tablespoons fresh basil
- One tablespoon fresh mint
- One apple
- Pure water as needed

Bring all ingredients into a container or mixer and shake or combine together. Makes dressing in 2/3 cups.

Garden Tonic

- A big handful of spinach
- One medium carrot
- Three stalks of celery

- Two stalks of asparagus

- One large tomato Water as needed

When you put together a juicer, juice spinach, carrot, and celery, followed by asparagus and tomato, pour all into one shot and enjoy it.

We can use a mixer if you do not have a juicer. Break the celery and asparagus into 1-2 inch sections crosswise. Bring the ingredients together in a blender. Cover and mix until well blended at high speed, adding water if appropriate. Garnish with a lemon wedge or cherry tomato.

Raspberry Coconut Slush

- Three tablespoons shredded unsweetened coconut

- 1/2 cup almonds (soaked overnight)

- Two tablespoons flax seeds (soaked overnight)

- One tablespoon psyllium seed

- half teaspoon ground cardamom (or other spice you prefer)

- two cups herb tea (brewed)

- one cup of pure water

- half cup raspberries fresh or frozen

Place the coconut, almonds, flax, psyllium, and cardamom in a food processor or blender and process sufficiently brewed tea. Blend until smooth. Add remaining tea, water, then raspberries, then start processing until dense and smooth. In the lakes serve. Then thin the tea further, and drink it. If you want a thicker, cooler result cover any water with ice.

3.7 Snacks and Handhelds

Dried Veggie Chips

- One medium eggplant, cut into thin slices

- One teaspoon sea salt

- One tablespoon extra-virgin olive oil

- Two teaspoons tamari

- Two zucchinis, cut diagonally into thin slices

- Two medium kohlrabies, peeled, halved and cut into thin slices one medium jicama, peeled and cut into thin slices

- One red bell pepper, cut into thin strips

Cut the eggplant, then mix with one tablespoon of sea salt and allow it to settle for about 30 minutes. Rinse, wipe.

Meanwhile, in a large pot, add olive oil and tamari. Add vegetables and cover with the toss. Place powdered slices on the dehydrator screens or on the baking sheet, which is lightly greased.

Dehydrate for 4-8 hours at 110 degrees F. Change the temperature to the lowest possible level when using an oven and steam for 3-4 hours until the vegetables are dried and leathery. It may take longer to get thicker slices and weathered vegetables (like zucchini).

Flax Crackers

- Four cups whole flax seeds soaked 4-6 hours

- 1/3 cup low-salt tamari

- Juice of three lemons

Soak the flax seeds in purified water for 4 to 6 hours. Pour out excess water.

Then you get a gelatinous blend. Stir in Braggs and lemon juice and mix properly. Keep wet and spread loosely.

Put the mixture evenly onto the dehydrator trays with a sheet of telex on top. Keep your hands moist as this will help spread the flax seeds at 105 degrees F (or use a spatula). Flip the mixture for 5-6 hours and remove the telex sheet. Attempt to dehydrate until the mixture is completely dry (about 5-6 hours)

Variation: Use some variation of garlic, onions, carrot juice, taco seasoning, Italian seasoning, chili powder, or cumin. Create your own vision and be creative.

Lettuce Roll-Ups

Use two large leaves of leafy or Romaine lettuce, washed and patted dry for each roll-up. Fill with any the following combinations. Roll leaves and a toothpick secures. Cover with wax paper, cover parchment or plastic wrap, and store in the fridge.

Mixture 1

- One avocado
- One orange
- Sprinkle of rice vinegar
- Half grapefruit

Mixture 2

- Water packed canned salmon or tuna
- half cucumber, finely chopped
- 1/4 red onion, finely chopped

Mixture 3

- half cup ground walnuts
- half cup apple, finely chopped Sprinkle of lemon juice

Mixture #4

- One red bell pepper, chopped fine
- One carrot, shredded
- 1 cup cabbage, finely shredded
- One stalk celery, minced

Mixture #5

- Four tablespoons pine nuts, chopped
- 1/2 cup chopped wild mushrooms
- 1/8 teaspoon flaked seaweed
- One carrot, shredded

Notes: Create your own Roll-ups Recipe. You can also use steamed cabbage leaves, if you like, instead of lettuce leaves.

You may want to use one of the sauces or dips from the Sauces and Dressings section of our Recipes to add different tastes or mouthfeel.

Sprout and Jicama Snack

Two cups mung bean sprouts

- One cup sunflower seed sprouts
- One cup lentil sprouts
- 1/8 cup radish sprouts
- 1/3 cup onion sprouts
- One cup additional mixed sprouts of your choice
- 1/2 cup grated jicama
- One tablespoon Salt-Free All-Purpose Seasoning*
- One teaspoon extra virgin olive oil
- One teaspoon Spike or seasoning

In a large bowl, combine the sprouts and jicama together. Brush the olive oil over the sprouts and mix well. Seasonings brush in.

Note: Try different forms of sprouts and their proportions various seasonings trial.

Vegetable Leather

- Four cups vegetables, your choice of any on the Recommended list, or 4 cups thick, vegetable soup

- One teaspoon tamari

- One teaspoon lemon juice

Vegetables made from steam. In a blender or food processor, mix well; then season with tamari and lemon juice. Put the pureed vegetable mixture in a food dehydrator on a Teflon tray and dehydrate at 135 degrees F for about 6 hours or until it is no longer sticky.

Lightly spray a cookie sheet when using an oven and pour puree over the tray. Cook until soft and leathery, at the lowest possible oven temperature.

Vegetable Wraps

- 2 cups flax seeds, ground 1

- 1/2 cups water

- One teaspoon Spike

- Three cloves garlic, peeled

- 1 cup fresh basil, chopped

- 1/2 cup fresh parsley, chopped

- 1/4 medium onion, chopped

- 1 cup sun-dried tomatoes

- Two red bell peppers, chopped

- 1/4 teaspoon cayenne pepper

- One teaspoons marjoram

- Two teaspoons lime juice

Grind the flax seeds to a fine meal in a spice or coffee grinder. Place all remaining ingredients in blender or food processor, except water and seed meal, and combine well.

Stir well in water and seed meal and set aside for at least 30 minutes or until the mixture has thickened. Drop onto Teflon dehydrator boards by the spoonful, spreading each cover into a thin circular shape.

Dehydrate to 105 F. Easily uninstall for 6 hours or until. Attach to the mesh sheets, and dry until leathery for a couple more hours.

Note: Use a tortilla just as you would. Pack in refrigerated plastic bags for up to 30 days. Earnings: 8 wrap

3.8 Sauces and Dressings

Asian Dressing

1 cup raw hulled (white) sesame seeds

- 1 cup brewed black tea

- One tablespoon rice vinegar

- 1/2 teaspoon chili flakes (optional)

- Two cloves garlic, chopped

- Two tablespoons tamari

- Two tablespoons fresh ginger

The sesame seeds are pounded to a fine meal in a coffee bean grinder or food processor. All ingredients Place in a blender and combine until smooth, adding as much water as necessary to achieve the desired consistency.

Balsamic Vinaigrette Dressing

One tablespoon extra-virgin oil

- 1/4 teaspoon tamari

- One teaspoon balsamic vinegar Fresh ground pepper to taste

- One teaspoon Dijon mustard

- Two teaspoons freshly squeezed lemon juice Dash of hot sauce

Blend all ingredients. Store in an airtight container in the refrigerator. Use on any salad.

BBQ Sauce

- 1 cup walnut or hemp oil

- 2 cups cider vinegar

- Two tablespoons poultry seasoning

- Three tablespoons Spike seasoning

- Half teaspoon black pepper (optional)One egg

Combine butter, vinegar then seasonings into a strong saucepan. Bring to boil, reduce heat, and cook for 5 minutes. Take off fire. Whisk in the beaten egg and let cool down. Place in a jar refrigerated with a lid. Keeps until 60 days.

Dijon Vinaigrette

- 1/2 cup extra virgin olive oil

- Two tablespoons red or white wine vinegar

- One teaspoon Dijon mustard

- One small shallot, minced (optional)

- A little salt and pepper

In blender or shaker, mix both ingredients with cap. Hold in a sealed jar, refrigerated. Can

Fines Herbs

- One tablespoon dried thyme

- One tablespoon dried savory

- One tablespoon dried marjoram

- One tablespoon dried sage

- One tablespoon dried basil

- One tablespoon dried grated lemon peel

Great Plant is a blend of various amounts of chopped aromatic herbs. The list cited above is just one example, and such herbs as parsley, chervil, tarragon, and chives may also be used. Sauces, beef, poultry, seafood, sautéed vegetables, soups, and omelets may be flavored with the mixture. Mix herbs and lemon peel. Store in an airtight container. Keep in a cool, dry place.

Ginger Dressing

One teaspoon grated ginger root

- Two tablespoons walnut oil

- Two shallots, finely chopped

- One teaspoon tamari

- Three tablespoons rice vinegar

Combine all ingredients in a jar. Cap and shake well.

Grapefruit Vinaigrette

- 1/4 cup freshly squeezed grapefruit juice

- 3/4 cup extra virgin olive oil

- One teaspoon, Spike, or Salt-Free All-Purpose Seasoning*

Blend and bottle. Keep refrigerated. The recipe can be doubled.

Green Salsa

- 4-7 jalapeno or Serrano chilies

- One clove garlic

- 1 pound tomatillos (husked)

- One ripe avocado

- 1/2 cup chopped cilantro

- One lime

- Morton Salt Substitute

The grill of roast chilies and tomatillos. In a blender, either add the garlic with a little water or scramble with a garlic press. Combine garlic with chilies, and tomatillos roasted and blend at low speed

Scramble, or thinly chip off the avocado. In a cup, mix avocado, cilantro, and blender milk. Squeeze lime over vinegar, and add salt or salt to taste.

Herb Dressing

- Two stalks celery and leaves, chopped fine

- Two small green onions, chopped fine

- Four sprigs parsley, chopped fine

- One teaspoon paprika

- 1/4 teaspoon dried basil

- 1/8 teaspoon marjoram or rosemary

- 1 cup olive oil

- 2/3 cup lemon juice

Add all the ingredients and mix them properly in the mixer. Enable to stay overnight in the refrigerator or until flavors are combined.

Herbs de Provence Spice Mix

Three tablespoons dried marjoram

- Three tablespoons dried thyme
- Three tablespoons dried savory
- One teaspoon dried basil
- One teaspoon dried rosemary
- 1/2 teaspoon dried sage
- 1/2 teaspoon fennel seeds

Combine all ingredients. Mix well and spoon into small jars. Use to season chicken, vegetables, or meat.

Italian Basil Pesto

- Two cups fresh basil leaves stemmed and packed
- 3/4 cup fresh parsley, chopped
- Half cup raw walnuts or pine nuts
- Two cloves garlic, peeled (use more if you wish)
- Half teaspoon grated lemon rind
- Half cup extra virgin olive oil
- Half teaspoons Morton Salt Substitute

Combine all ingredients in a blender and heat until fairly smooth. Put in the freezer. This will last for up to three weeks.

Latin Salsa

- Six cloves garlic, peeled
- Three to five Serrano chilies
- one cup cilantro
- Juice of 1 lime

- 3-4 tomatillos, outer husks removed (or use two more tomatoes instead)

- 3-4 medium tomatoes

- One teaspoon ground cumin

- One medium-large red onion, chopped into 1/4 pieces

A blender is an ideal instrument for salsa development. To create a chunky texture, apply ingredients in the order specified below to the blender, and do not over-mix at the last. Mix enough to split the last few tomatoes, but not so much to pulverize them.

In a blender, place the garlic, chilies, cilantro, and lime juice. Repeated pulse blender until garlic is a paste and finely chopped chilies and cilantro leaves. If required, scrape down the sides of the blender.

If the mixture is too dry to properly handle, add a few tomatillos, or a tomato. Remove remaining tomatillos and pulse them to break. Then add tomatoes and cumin and pulse the tomatoes just enough to crack. Measure the salsa into a saucepan.

Manually add the onion into the salsa. Let the salsa stand as the flavors mix for an hour. Refrigerate then in a sealed jar.

Lemon Mint Dressing

Five tablespoons extra virgin olive oil

- Three tablespoons lemon or lime juice

- Two tablespoons white vinegar

- One clove garlic, minced

- 1/2 teaspoon dried mint (or one teaspoon fresh mint, minced)

- 1/2 teaspoon dried basil

Put all ingredients into a container or mixer and shake or combine together. Makes dressing in 2/3 cups.

Lemon Vinaigrette

- A dash of seasoning

- 3/4 cup extra virgin olive oil

- One teaspoon parsley (fresh or dried), or any fresh herbs you like (rosemary, savory, thyme, dill, sage, etc.)

- 1/4 cup freshly squeezed lemon

Blend and store in a bottle. Keep refrigerated. The recipe can be doubled.

Lime, Oil and Garlic Dressing

- 1-2 teaspoons tamari

- One teaspoon garlic, peeled and finely chopped

- finely chopped of Two tablespoons shallots,

- less than half cup lime juice, plus extra if needed

- One cup extra-virgin olive oil and extra if needed Freshly ground black pepper

Whisk tamari, tomatoes, and shallots and lime juice in a small bowl. Whisk slowly in the oil until it emulsifies.

Seasonings taste and change, adding more lime juice if appropriate pack overnight in an airtight container, or until well-blended flavors.

Mango Salsa

- One ripe mango, diced

- One papaya, diced

- 1/2 medium red onion, chopped

- 1 Serrano or jalapeño chili pepper (or use milder Anaheim), minced (optional)

- One small cucumber diced

- Two tablespoons fresh cilantro leaves, chopped

- Three tablespoons fresh lime juice and Pepper to taste

All ingredients Place in a bowl and mix well. Let salsa stand at room temperature for one hour to allow flavors to blend. Hot in a sealed container.

Meat Marinade No. 1

- One tablespoon honey

- Half cup olive oil

- Four cloves garlic, crushed

- 1/4 cup tamari

- Two teaspoons rice vinegar

Put all the ingredients in a small bowl and whisk until well combined. Put meat or poultry into a bag with a zip lock. Sprinkle in the marinade. Refrigerate, if you have time, then leave overnight. Otherwise, leave it to marinate for 1 to 4 hours

Remove the meat and go about frying or bbq. Before frying, put some of the marinades on top of the meat. Once you turn the meat over, just based on another bone. When barbecue, often based on meat to keep it moist.

Meat Marinade No. 2

- One tablespoon honey

- 1/2 cup olive oil

- Three tablespoons lime juice

- Two teaspoons fresh ginger root, finely grated

- 1/4 cup tamari

Same instructions as above.

Mexican Guacamole

Two avocados

- One onion, chopped fine

- One tomato, chopped fine

- 1-2 limes or one lemon, juiced (to taste)

- Two cloves garlic, minced

- One tablespoon cilantro, minced

- One jalapeno chopped

Break avocados in two, pick the flesh out with a knife, or place them in a food processor or blender, depending on whether you like your smooth or chunky guacamole

Place all ingredients in bowl and mix, including lemon or lime juice. Stir in lemon or lime juice and mix again

Variation: Take Mexican Guacamole and mix some with a different taste and texture of any salsa dish.

Mock Sour Cream

- One cup Brazil nuts, soaked overnight

- 1/4 cup lemon juice

- Half teaspoon tamari

Apply 1/3 cup of water to a blender or food processor. Combine the almonds, lemon juice, and tamari for about 3 to 4 minutes, until light and creamy. Add more water, if needed.

Variation: Substitute lemon juice with lime juice and apply cumin and chili powder to taste. Use another nut or crop, if you want to.

Mushroom Gravy

- Half cup soaked almonds
- Half cup organic beef broth (use more if needed)
- Two cups shitake mushrooms (use another mushroom if shitake not available)
- 1/4 teaspoon garlic granules or one clove garlic
- Two teaspoons tamari

Blend the almonds and the beef broth together until smooth; set aside. Combine mushrooms with just enough beef broth to get the gravy consistency needed.

Blend in coconut, garlic, tamari, and seasonings. Again blend until smooth, adding more broth if needed. Heat up, then drink.

Nut Pâté

- One cup walnuts
- Half cup almonds
- Half cup macadamia nuts
- 1/4 cup sesame seeds
- One red bell pepper, finely chopped
- Three stalks celery, finely chopped
- One small leek (white part only), finely chopped
- Two tablespoons lemon juice
- one to two teaspoons powdered kelp
- One or two tablespoons tamari

Soak all the nuts and seeds in pure water for 12-24 hours, then rinse. I use a food processor, grind all the nuts and seeds until they have been reduced to a meal.

Add pepper with the red bell, celery, leek, lemon juice, kelp, tamari, and blend well.

Olive Oil-Lemon Dressing

- Three tablespoons fresh-squeezed lemon juice
- Half cup olive oil (may also use flax, walnut or hemp)
- One clove garlic, peeled
- Herb seasoning for taste

Herb seasoning ideas: Oregano-for a more Italian Flavor Thyme-for a moderate herbal Basil flavor-for a heavy herbal Cayenne flavor-for those who like spicy food shake all the ingredients in a bottle with a tight-fitting lid. Keep relaxing.

When olive oil solidifies, draw one hour before using it from the refrigerator. Use vegetable or salad dishes.

Omega 3 Mayonnaise

- One tablespoon lemon juice
- One whole egg
- 1/4 teaspoon dry mustard
- 1/3 cup olive oil
- 1/3 cup flaxseed oil
- 1/3 cup walnut oil

In a blender, place the lemon juice, potato, and mustard blend 3 to 5 seconds. Start blending and add oils gradually while the blender is on low in a thin stream. Blend until thick with mayonnaise. Put in a plastic sealed container. Usage in 5-7 days' time.

Note: If both flaxseed oil and walnut oil do not exist, use 2/3 cup of the one you have. Rent: 1 cup

Pork Loin Marinade

- 1/4 pineapple
- One orange
- 2-3 tablespoons olive oil
- 1/3 - 1/2 cup tamari
- One teaspoon ground ginger
- One small onion, chopped
- Two cloves garlic, minced

Break the pineapple outer skin away and peel an orange. Puree pineapple and orange in a blender or food processor.

In a jar with a tight-fitting lid, combine all ingredients. Shake well. Pour over meat. In the refrigerator, marinate, occasionally turning, for several hours or overnight before cooking.

Salt-Free All-Purpose Seasoning

- 1/4 cup dried minced onion
- Four teaspoon dried vegetable flakes
- One tablespoon garlic powder
- One tablespoon dried orange peel
- One teaspoon dried lemon peel
- 1-2 teaspoons coarse ground black pepper (optional)
- One teaspoon dried parsley
- Half teaspoon dried basil
- Half teaspoon dried marjoram
- half teaspoon dried oregano
- Half teaspoon dried savory
- Half teaspoon dried thyme

- Half teaspoon cayenne pepper (optional)
- Half teaspoon cumin
- Half teaspoon coriander
- Half teaspoon dried mustard 1/4 teaspoon celery seed

Two teaspoons dried Nori flakes

In a grinder, mix all the ingredients and grind to a paste. Place the spice mix in a sealed shaker jar or closed bag.

Spicy Salad Dressing

- Six tablespoons extra virgin olive oil
- Two tablespoons lemon juice
- One teaspoon dry oregano
- One teaspoon dried parsley
- 1/2 teaspoon curry powder
- One clove garlic, peeled and minced
- Dash of Salt-Free All-Purpose Seasoning and Dash of freshly ground black pepper

Mix all ingredients and let them rest for at least 10 minutes. Add to any salad. Top with avocado, onion, and tomato.

Tapenade

- Six tablespoons walnuts or pine nuts
- Two cloves garlic, peeled and pressed
- One green onion (white part only)
- Half cup Italian parsley stemmed and chopped
- One cup fresh spinach stemmed and chopped
- 1/4 fresh thyme
- Half teaspoon grated lemon peel

- Half teaspoon Morton Salt Substitute or 1/8 teaspoon regular salt

- 3/4 cup black olives, pitted

- Three tablespoons extra virgin olive oil

In the food processor, place nuts and garlic and process until the nuts are crushed. Add onion, parsley, spinach, and thyme and thoroughly process.

Add salt, lemon peel, and olive oil and blend until smooth. Turn to the box, and store in the fridge.

Tartar Sauce

- 1 cup Omega 3 mayonnaise*

- Two tablespoons red onion, finely chopped

- 1/2 tablespoon lime or lemon juice

- 1/2 teaspoon dried dill

- 1/4 teaspoon paprika

- 1/2 tablespoon Dijon mustard

- One tablespoon drained capers

- One tablespoon cucumber, peeled and finely chopped

Put Omega 3 mayonnaise into a bowl. Add all ingredients and whisk until mixed. Serve straight away or refrigerate 2-3 days in a sealed container.

Tomato Chili Salsa

- One clove garlic, peeled and minced

- One pound tomatoes, chopped small

- Half cup bell, Anaheim or Serrano peppers, chopped

- Half small red onion, finely chopped

- 1/4 cup fresh cilantro, finely chopped

- 1/4 cup fresh parsley, finely chopped

- One tablespoon lime juice

- One teaspoon white vinegar

- Half teaspoon Spike seasoning

Mix cabbage, cilantro, parsley, lime juice, vinegar, and seasonings of onions, tomatoes, peppers. Fill with plastic food wrap, and let stay at room temperature for 1 hour. Keeps an average of 10 days in the fridge.

Variation: RED HOT SALSA: raise the garlic to 2 cloves, add the lime juice to 1/2 spoonful's and add one spoonful of chopped jalapeno pepper, plus 1/4 teaspoon red pepper. Continue as laid out above.

Chapter 4: PCOS Dietary Tips

4.1 Eat Organic

Organic foods provide two main benefits: Less in chemicals and other environmentally friendly products.

They have a high level of nutrients compared with non-organic foods.277 For reasons we addressed in What Causes PCOS, it is very important for you to reduce your exposure to environmental and other chemical substances and toxins?

You may take an important step towards reducing your exposure by moving to organic foods. Organic food is produced without the use of pesticides, artificial fertilizers, or other chemicals.

Food pesticides are potentially your main concern. To order to increase crop yields, improve the appearance of food, and increase profits, many crops are heavily sprayed with pesticides. Chemical pesticides are not only bug-toxic but poisonous to you as well.

As pesticides and other chemicals are applied to food crops, some of the chemicals are ingested directly from the spray while others are absorbed from the ground through the plant's roots into the plant.

Although the U.S. is banned or restricted on the use of certain pesticides such as DDT, many of our products are imported from countries outside the United States, which have little or no restrictions on the use of pesticides on plants. Products from other nations are far more likely than products from the United States to produce higher levels of pesticides.

Since the difference between domestic and foreign goods is nearly impossible to tell, you might be exposed to more pesticides than you think. This is a strong reason for choosing organic food.

Organic Foods Free of Pesticides

However, organic foods contain only 1/10 more than a pesticide as prone to residues. A new study of 94, samples of foods has shown that organic foods (not including pesticide use) often contain pesticides but only 1/3 more than traditional foods.

A large proportion of pesticide residues in organic food come from long-lasting yet eco-hardened chemical products like DDT, which plants will absorb from the atmosphere years after farmers avoid using them. Pesticides may also have migrated from a non-organic field into an organic field.

Almost all of our food, water, and air are polluted. Your aim is to do your best to reduce your visibility. Organic products have lower pesticide levels and higher nutrient levels than conventional products.

Grow Your Own Vegetables

The best way to eat healthily is through the production of your own plants.

We strongly recommend that you start your own organic vegetable garden if you have space and time. It offers some significant advantages:

You can eat food picked minutes or hours earlier. The majority of products on the market are several days to weeks old and have lost much of their most delicate nutrients.

- Organic growth of nutrients is much richer.
- Working in your garden is enjoyable, a good workout, and a way to relieve stress.

- You are happy to create some of the food you eat.

4.2 Eating in Restaurants

You are in trouble if you often eat in restaurants. Research by the University of Tufts found that those who ate food more often than not were overweight and reversing it was leaner people who ate food from restaurants.

More often than not, those who eat restaurant food consumed more calories and fat and less fiber than those who eat less often restaurant food.

For instance, restaurant foods have 18 percent higher intakes of calories per kilogram, 12 percent higher in total fat, and 36 percent lower in fiber compared to restaurant foods that have consumed fewer than 4.3 times a month. Nutrition in the restaurant 13 times a month versus 4.3 times a month was equal to about 5 percent of body fat. According to this report, a 5% weight loss may result from the simple avoidance of restaurants.

And we're not living in a perfect universe. Often, you are going to eat out. Every chapter offers advice on how the meal can be made healthier.

Restaurant Food Selection

Provide some carbohydrates in the meal, such as grilled salmon, to reduce the blood sugar fluctuations. Evite high-glycemic carbohydrates, including pasta, crackers, baked potatoes, and white rice. Have then a salad and a platter of vegetables.

Be sure there is no MSG (monosodium glutamate) in your meal. If you're in a Chinese or Japanese bar, make sure to ask.

The part of the meal you are served may be much bigger than you like. Feed only gradually when you're done leaving something on your plate.

A few guidelines are listed below when dining out in restaurants. They're not "ideal" suggestions, but they send you some guidance, at least.

Soup & Salad Restaurant

Avoid

- Frozen yogurt, puddings, whipped cream

- Pizza

- Salad dressings that have oil

- Margarine, butter and butter spreads

- Muffins and bread

Preferred Choices

- Olive oil for salad dressing

- The fat things are grouped in separate areas, so you can easily avoid them

- Cafeteria-style (you get to control the choice of food)

Seafood Restaurant

Avoid

- Deep-fried seafood

- Seafood dunked in butter or batter

- Combination plates, which usually have something fried

- Stuffed seafood

Preferred Choices

- Clear seafood gumbo is better than creamy seafood bisque

- Manhattan clam chowder is better than the creamy New England version.

- Poached or grilled seafood is better than fried

- Lemon juice better is better than tartar

- Poached fish with vegetables and salad.

American Steak House

Avoid

- all cuts of red meat

- Ribs

- White rice

Avoid

Everything

Preferred Choices

- Grilled chicken

- London broil

- Focus on salad and vegetables

Preferred Choices

- Roast turkey

- Grilled chicken

- Soups, although they may be too salty

- dressing on the side and Tossed salad

- Steamed vegetables

Pizza Place

Avoid

·Everything

Preferred Choices

·Salad

Delicatessen

Avoid

· Everything

Preferred Choices

- Some delis have good soups
- Roast turkey

Mexican Restaurant

Avoid

- Deep-fried corn tortillas
- sour cream or Cheese
- Go easy on the refried beans

Preferred Choices

- Guacamole
- Soup
- Chicken or fish taco
- Salad

Chinese Restaurant

Avoid

- Stay away from any food that has MSG
- White steamed rice
- Fried rice
- Egg rolls
- Fried wontons
- Fried noodles
- Most meat dishes
- Sweet and sour dishes
- Most Chinese food

Preferred Choices

- Chop suey better than chow Mein

- Stir-fried dishes in moderation
- Some seafood dishes
- Some vegetable dishes

Salad Dressings

Avoid

- Cheesy
- Creamy

Preferred Choices

- Vinegar & herb
- Salsa
- Oil-free dressing

Entrée

Avoid

- Gravies or sauces on the entree
- Deep-fried

Better Choices

- Roasted, baked, broiled, boiled
- Cut all visible fat
- Remove skin from poultry
- Sauces served on the side

Vegetables

Avoid

- Served in a cream or sauce
- Deep-fried and breaded

Preferred Choices

- Stewed

- Steamed
- Boiled
- Baked
- Raw

Breakfast

Avoid

- Bacon
- Ham
- Hash browns
- Omelets
- Fried eggs
- Eggs Benedict

Better Choices

- Poached or hardboiled egg
- Low-fat cottage cheese (if necessary)
- Vegetable side dish if available
- Hot oatmeal (not instant)

Beverages

Avoid

- Ice
- Coffee
- Milk
- Soft drinks
- Fruit juice or fruit drinks

Better Choices

- Water Also add a slice of lemon for flavor

- Mineral or sparkling water

- Tomato, V8 or other vegetable juice

- Tea

Desserts

Avoid

· There are no healthy prepared desserts

Better Choices

- A small amount of fresh fruit (not melon)

- The small number of raw nuts or seeds - ask your server, they may have some on hand

Food Safety

When dining out, try eating only food that was prepared right before you were served. Ask your server if your food is ready and freshly cooked is a good idea. To order to save money, some restaurants have food prepared in advance by external suppliers or store food for too long without throwing it out. As a consequence, pathogenic bacteria can be infected.

Soups, sauces, and stews are kept in large, often uncovered containers in some restaurants and delicacies for easy microwave heating while ordering. Cooking with microwaves may not kill salmonella or other pathogenic bacteria strains.

Be cautious about salad bars. At first glance, salad bars appear to be a good place to eat healthily. Yet look again. Look again. The Wall Street Journal sent out a writer a few years ago to investigate the cleanliness of salad bars in various parts of the world. Problems with both the restaurant and the clientele were seen. In their use of salad bars, people are unhealthy. Often the sample and replenish food. The handles of the serving utensils often slip in the food trays and are contaminated.

Do not eat food that a street vendor has prepared. You have no way of assessing food safety.

Remove restaurants with flies. Flies will disperse parasite cysts and pathogenic bacteria and show that cleanliness does not bother the owner.

4.3 Eating Away from Home

Many people are on their way, whether for a company or social reasons. Here are some tips and suggestions when you are away from home.

Eating in the Office

The best way is by far to carry your lunch home. In this way, you have complete control over what you eat.

You should carry leftovers from dinner last night (such as salmon, salad and vegetables). Or take home-made soups, including vegetable and beef soup.

Take a piece of fresh fruit and chocolate nuts. Instead of coffee or soft drinks, you can have herbal tea, green tea, or sparkling water.

Parties

If you go to a party without a sit-down, we recommend you have a meal before you go home.

The preferred drinks will be if you want to consume alcohol, beer, or wine. Hard liquor is not recommended. However, if you plan to drink hard liquor, please take a B-complex tablet and a multivitamin tablet in advance to help the body maintain healthy blood sugar.

Eat as many vegetables as you want at the party. Check for fresh fruit if vegetables are not available. Stay away from crackers, potato chips, and other junk food. Stay away.

Take part in discussions and try to keep the food at least six feet away. Drink lots of non-alcoholic drinks, including sparkling water.

Visiting

When it comes to food, visiting a family or a friend can be a touching thing. Tell your host in advance that you have a special diet and will not be able to enjoy his delicious desserts and fried foods.

If you have a specially prepared fatty, sugar-packaged or high-glycemic food, just leave some (or more) on your plates.

If you learn that the host doesn't have enough food in the house in advance, try to cook and bring a nutritious meal. And offer to bring some healthy ingredients and help your host prepare the meal with the ingredients.

Don't panic if your host gives you pancakes, fried eggs, and English breakfast muffins. Have breakfast, and enjoy the conversation. You don't have to eat all on your plate.

On the Road

Hotels

It is sometimes difficult to get food or eat a meal somewhere. You can, therefore, have to plan ahead.

Prepare and bring healthy snacks to your house. For starters, you can bring a few apples and nuts.

Or you could bring a high-protein meal replacement powder with you and a plastic shake mixer. Add water or perhaps some fruit juice (50/50 water-diluted) and yogurt. Play together and relax. Relax.

Another option is to stop in your health center to have healthy snacks. If there's no convenient food store, go to a large supermarket to find something good.

See if the hotel offers a buffet at breakfast. Look over; you may find that it helps you to choose food better than on the menu. In any case, a fair breakfast would include hot oatmeal, eggs, and your option of drink (not orange juice).

Most hotels offer a fantastic buffet lunch, including a salad bar, a soup bar, and a hot menu. Have a few chicken or fish along with a few vegetable dishes and perhaps a salad.

Keep it light for dinner, particularly if it's late. An option is sliced turkey or fish with steamed vegetables. Or a bowl of chicken.

In Your Car

The planning before you leave your journey is the secret to healthy eating! Shop at a convenience store to guarantee that you eat poor quality food. Prepare a variety of snacks before you leave. Bring a small cooler if you have to stay cold.

When you plan to go camping, fill your cooler with several pre-cooked or ready meals to make it easy and healthy for your camp to eat.

On-Campus

You have little to know about what is available when you stay in a college dorm or boarding or sorority house where food is prepared for yourselves. Your options are even less than in a restaurant. For refined carbohydrates, the most' institutional' food is too big, which is exactly the type of food that you want to avoid.

If you have a meal, have animal protein and vegetables. Minimize the amount of grain and avoid all baked goods. Don't have a snack except for fresh fruit.

In some cases, workers will prepare food for people with special needs, including diabetics. If your staff should cook special meals, show the workers relevant parts of this book and see if they are able to prepare food that complies with our guidelines.

If the food you eat does not provide you with enough high-quality protein, then you might be able to make protein shakes in your house, even without a refrigerator. You could have a mixer, a whey protein concentrate protein powder, and fresh fruit in hand, for example. You may blend protein powder, water, and fresh fruit as a snack or meal substitute. Another way to have a meal in a restaurant or at a friend's house on occasion.

4.4 Healthy Eating Habits

How you eat is the most important thing. But improving your health regarding how you eat is also very important. The development of the best physical and emotional atmosphere helps you digest and consume the food you eat. It also reduces possible rises in the stress hormone cortisol, which causes problems for PCOS patients.

- Meditate briefly or at least take a deep breath to relax before you start eating.
- Do not read the newspaper, watch television, or think about bad food.
- Eat slowly. Slowly. If you don't rush, you can eat less and enjoy your meal more. Slowly feeding always increases the digestion.
- Chew your food well. Chew your food well. Don't eat it if you can't chew it well.
- Complete what you chew before you put more food in your mouth.
- Do not feed again after eating until food is digested.

- Avoid foods that cause discomfort, no matter how safe they are supposed to be. You may be allergic or intolerant.
- Do not drink ice water or cold meal beverages. The cold slows digestion.
- Don't feed when in pain, emotionally upset, exhausted, or after hard work immediately.
- Eat food below room temperature (not cool, not steam piped).
- Drink less than you thought. If you're not sure that you had enough, wait 5-10 minutes before you decide to eat more.
- Don't skip breakfast, don't forget it. Feed around 4-5 times a day. The blood sugar is more regulated.
- Every time you eat, have some protein. It balances your blood sugar.
- The cleaning of your teeth will make your mouth feel like food and will warn you that you will no longer eat food for a while. If the weather is good, go around the block or indulge in some other activity to take away the dessert or eat more food from your mind.

When you should eat

Other women who stress about their weight or lead a busy life will often skip breakfast and don't each have a lot during the day. But they have a big dinner and snack in the evening when they come home. You don't want to do that!

Have Breakfast

Evidence suggests that a high-quality breakfast protein consumption can help balance leptin, maintain weight and energy, and help you regulate appetite during the day. A blend of protein, starch, fat, and fiber should be used.

You may find that in the morning, particularly if you are used to skipping breakfast, you are not hungry.

We encourage you to have breakfast anyway. When you start having breakfast regularly, you can grow the habit of eating more calories earlier in the day.

Note that you are most busy during the day and are most likely to burn calories instead of storing them. So the time to bring calories on board is not later than earlier in the day.

Meal Frequency

While there is some variation, most doctors recommend that people with blood sugar issues consume fewer, more frequent foods.

In this scenario, you would consider having breakfast, a snack in the mid-morning, lunch, a snack, and dinner in the afternoon. You would have a small snack in the evening only if necessary and if you are not overweight.

If you eat three, four, five, or six times a day, try to eat regularly. A survey of ten overweight women at Nottingham University, UK. It has shown that regular meals have resulted in slightly decreased calorie intake, reduced meal insulin, reduced cholesterol, and increased calorie burning.281 Moreover, pick your meal snacks carefully in between. These should be low and, as far as possible, avoid refined, processed foods. The Goteborg University study in Sweden has shown that overweight people do not snack more than normal people but prefer sweet fatty foods. In other words, snacking is all right as long as you avoid fattening, unhealthy foods.

Dinnertime

Dinner is not expected to be the day's biggest meal. Most likely, after dinner, you'll be inactive and then go to bed. A few of the calories you eat are burned away by physical activity, so a big, calorie-laden meal and late evening snacks are not required.

4.5 Tips for Increasing Your Fertility

Here are some easy nutritional tips to improve your likelihood of becoming pregnant.

Stop the Junk Food

Junk food is food that is high in calories but nutritionally low. Such calories are known as in empty calories.' Of refined carbohydrates, sweeteners, and poor quality fats, junk foods are typically high. These are packed and presented attractively and are easy to eat. They taste good, too.

Look at the label before consuming some highly prepared food and think, "Do I really have to consume it?"

Eat Whole Foods

The converse is to increase the consumption of whole foods by avoiding junk foods. Entire foods are the basis of this book's recipes. Whole foods provide you with the dietary elements to bring the hormones closer to normal and to be productive.

Whole foods are not refined. What would you like when you went to a friend's home, and she gave you a glass of apple juice, a cup of coffee, or an egg? Even if the apple juice or applesauce were more enticing, you'd choose the fruit. The apple is the best food bang for the buck.

Wherever possible, pick whole foods, regardless of where you are or what you are doing.

Go Organic

Enormous amounts of chemical waste are applied to our atmosphere every year. Some of them end up naturally in our food supply. Almost all of these compounds are poisonous to the body, and some are' hormone imitators' or' hormone disorders,' which can reduce fertility.

Monoculture has also drained our nitrogen soils. Food can look the same but contains lower amounts of nutrients.

Through buying organic foods or cultivating some of your own foods, you will mitigate these problems.

Avoid Genetically Modified Foods

In the last few decades, plants have been genetically modified to increase crop yields and to boost their production and marketing properties. This improves food producers, processors, and distributors ' income. You can rest assured that GM foods have not been produced to improve your health.

Genetically modified plants on a really massive scale have been introduced. It's too early to know if your fertility will be impacted by these food changes. Until the food industry can show that GM foods don't mess with your fertility, it's best to prevent them.

Balance Your Essential Fats

EFA is imbalanced (essential fatty acids) in people who eat a "new" diet of processed food. Such fats are important because you can't live without them and you have to eat them. The main fats are two groups: omega-6 and omega-3. Many people consume too much omega-6 and almost too little omega-3.

It will be almost hard for your hormone to get back on the track so that you can conceive before you regain this nutritional balance.

Minimize Gluten Grains

Gluten intolerant is a wide section of the population, which is mainly found in wheat, rye, and barley. Many people with gluten intolerance have deficits in infertility.

Wheat is by far the largest gluten source, like wheat, which is used in almost all baked goods and thousands of processed foods. The effect of gluten may be indirect because it damages the lining of the bowels and thus decreases food absorption of essential nutrients. Gluten itself can cause an unwanted immune response.

Have Plenty of Fiber

For optimum hormone excretion (such as estrogens) through stool. It also reduces food intake, so that blood sugar is more stable.

When we eat whole grains, we get all the nutrients you need. We may need to add additional fiber to your diet if you consume refined or processed foods. Adding fiber to a refined diet is not almost as effective as simply eating whole foods.

The diet high in saturated animal fats tends to increase oestrogen.

Reduce Saturated Fat

Women with PCOS may already have too high levels of estrogen compared to progesterone, which makes it difficult for them to ovulate.

A diet too high in saturated fats often inhibits the metabolism of EFAs (essential fatty acids), which produce disorderly cell function, which perpetuates hormonal imbalances.

Women in common "low carb" diets can eat too much-saturated fat to lose weight.

Change Your Carbs

Change Your Note that we haven't said: "carbs cut." "Increase the carbs," we said. You will recover fertility faster if you get rid of refined carbohydrates and focus more on unprocessed carbs.

Unprocessed carbs can be found mostly in whole vegetables and fruits, as well as in nuts and seeds. These are also present in grains and legumes, but we suggest that you restrict their intake.

In almost all packaged, manufactured foodstuffs, you will find unhealthy carbs.

Reduce Alcohol

If you seek to conceive of alcohol, studies suggest that you can increase your fertility by cutting your alcohol consumption drastically.

Reduce Stress

Stress hormones inhibit other hormones, including the hormones for reproduction. These also cause you to gain weight and make resistance to insulin worse. Concentrate on rising stress factors in your life to become fertile.

Exercise

Decreases resistance to insulin lowers body fat and provides many other health benefits. For most PCOS women, regular exercise will boost fertility.

Lose Weight

You will lose fat weight if you follow the above advice. It is hard to say how much weight you lose, but studies show a 5 percent -10 percent reduction in weight significantly improves the potential to get pregnant.

Reduce Insulin Resistance

As the resistance to insulin decreases, your testosterone should also decline, and your reproductive hormones will develop an acceptable relationship to enable you to ovulate and become pregnant.

Is your partner fertile?

Don't let your friend forget. Don't let your wife down. The reproduction of many mammals on Earth, including humans, has declined significantly in the last 60 years or so.

Men's and women's fertility has decreased. Male sperm count and motility dropped dramatically.

If you couldn't conceive but are ovulating, it would be prudent to have your husband test his sperm for quantity and viability.

Consider Nutritional Supplements

One way to help you guide the balance of your hormones in the right direction. For example, a significant number of supplements increase the sensitivity to insulin to a certain degree. There are many other foods that can help specifically control the reproductive hormones.

Consult a licensed health care professional knowing nutritional supplements and how they can be used to improve the hormone function and increase your fertility rates.

Conclusion

One of the most common diseases affecting reproductive-age women is PCOS. It has multiple components as a disorder, including behavioral, metabolic, and neurological, including long-term health complications that exceed life span.

On a higher-protein, lower-carbohydrate diet, some women lose more weight and feel better but the study is not definitive. Researchers have found a low-calorie, low-fat meal replacement lifestyle to be successful for some people, but there is no perfect diet for everyone.

In fact, when PCOS diet trials were tested by Researchers, they observed that the symptoms of PCOS improved on any diet that the women followed.

A food plan that contains plenty of plant foods (vegetables, bananas, nuts, legumes) along with good fats, balanced lean proteins, and low-fat dairy or calcium-rich dairy alternatives is certainly a good beginning.

What matters is to choose the best diet option that you should stick to — not just lose weight.

So find a Recipes you like — and make sure you get plenty of support to help you stick with it, as that's the key to success.

The best way to manage PCOS is through developing good food experiences through a healthy lifestyle, a good diet, and regular exercise.

References

- Campbell, K. and Campbell, K. (n.d.). *3 Day PCOS Meal Plan, Recipes, & Shopping List*. [online] Smart Fertility Choices. Available at: **https://www.smartfertilitychoices.com/pcos-diet-plan/**.

- PCOS Nutrition Center. (n.d.). *Recipes Archives - PCOS Nutrition Center*. [online] Available at: **https://www.pcosnutrition.com/category/recipes/**.

- Pinterest. (n.d.). *39 Best Morgan's pcos recipes images | Food recipes, Cooking recipes, Food*. [online] Available at: **https://www.pinterest.com/amyocker/morgans-pcos-recipes/**.

- EatingWell. (n.d.). *What Is a Healthy PCOS Diet?*. [online] Available at: **http://www.eatingwell.com/article/290695/what-is-a-healthy-pcos-diet/**.

- PCOS Personal Trainer. (n.d.). *Recipes for a PCOS-Friendly Holiday Feast*. [online] Available at: **https://pcospersonaltrainer.com/articles/pcos-holiday-recipes/**.

- Tarladalal.com. (n.d.). *PCOS Diet, PCOS recipes, Poly Cystic Ovary Syndrome Indian recipes*. [online] Available at: **https://www.tarladalal.com/recipes-for-PCOS-1040**.

- Martha McKittrick Nutrition. (n.d.). *Free PCOS Meal Plans and Recipes | Martha McKittrick Nutrition*. [online] Available at: **https://www.marthamckittricknutrition.com/free-pcos-meal-plans-and-recipes/**.